28 DAYS TO A BETTER BODY

A FOOD AND FITNESS PLAN FOR HEALTH

BY JANET THOMSON

≡People's Medical Society.

Allentown, Pennsylvania

The People's Medical Society is a nonprofit consumer health organization dedicated to the principles of better, more responsive and less expensive medical care. Organized in 1983, the People's Medical Society puts previously unavailable medical information into the hands of consumers so that they can make informed decisions about their own health care.

Membership in the People's Medical Society is $20 a year and includes a subscription to the *People's Medical Society Newsletter*. For information, write to the People's Medical Society, 462 Walnut Street, Allentown, PA 18102, or call 610-770-1670.

This and other People's Medical Society publications are available for quantity purchase at discount. Contact the People's Medical Society for details.

Library of Congress Cataloging-in-Publication Data

Thomson, Janet.
    28 days to a better body / Janet Thomson.
        p.   cm.
    Includes index.
    ISBN 1-882606-64-7
    1. Weight loss. 2. Health. I. Title.
    RM222.2.T4854   1995
    613.2'5 — dc20   96–13214
                                              CIP

First published in Great Britain by Thorsons, an imprint of HarperCollins Publishers Ltd., under the title *Fat to Flat*.

© 1995 by Janet Thomson

First published in the United States in 1996 by People's Medical Society.

1 2 3 4 5 6 7 8 9 0

First printing, September 1996
Text illustrations by Andrea Norton

Contents

Introduction

If you are serious about wanting to lose fat, then this is definitely the book for you! In it you will find lots of information about your body—how it works and what it needs to survive—as well as how to lose fat safely and effectively—*for good*.

In this day and age, there is a lot of pressure to conform to certain images of ultraskinny women or lean, muscular men. As a result of this, many "normal" people feel inadequate and unhappy about the way they look. We have become so concerned with how we look that we are prepared to go to almost any length to try to achieve the body beautiful—something that for most of us is unachievable. Inevitably this leads to disappointment. Everyone I know would like to change the look of some body part, and that includes me! Unfortunately many people abuse their bodies through months or even years of poor diets, often without realizing it. They follow the latest fad diet, taken in by false promises and expectations. Even though some of these diets result in drastic weight loss in a relatively short period of time, they can be very dangerous. As soon as you finish the diet, you start to regain the weight you lost, and often lots more besides.

Regaining weight has a very negative effect on your satisfaction with your appearance, your self-esteem and your confidence. It usually occurs because you were not on a well-balanced diet, and your body wasn't getting the amount of food it needed to stay healthy while you were on the plan. Or it may occur because you didn't prepare yourself for coping with high-risk situations. We all need to learn how to cope with temptation, and although this aspect of weight loss is often neglected, it is crucial to your long-term success. (See Chapter 3.)

In this book one of the most important things you will learn is how to set realistic goals. You will lose fat if you follow the guidelines set out in this book, but there will be no overnight change in how you look. Just as it takes a long time to become overweight, it can take a long time to lose weight safely, so that it stays off—for good.

So what are you expecting as you start to read this book? If you are hoping for an instant, 28-day miracle, you will be disappointed. My hope for you is that as you read you will learn to make changes in your life, in what you eat and in your activity levels, and that you will drastically improve your health. This has to be first and foremost. The wonderful thing about this book is that in addition to becoming healthier, you will also lose excess fat from your body. (That is, provided you actually follow the guidelines in this book—it's not enough just to read it!)

As you read you will learn that by reeducating yourself you can become healthier and slimmer at the same time. The majority of dieters feel anything from mild apprehension to dread at the thought of going on another diet. How do you feel as you are reading this? You can rest assured that this book *really* is different. I'm not trying to sell you some miracle food or potion that will solve all your problems. I have looked at weight loss from every angle, not just at what you put in your mouth—a successful weight-loss program has to offer much more than that. I will tell you how and why you gain fat, why your body naturally changes shape as you get older, exactly what your nutritional requirements are and why many diets simply can't work. I will explain why exercise is so important and how to choose the best forms of exercise for you. We will also look at the psychology of dieting (Why do we do it?), what you can realistically expect to achieve and, most important of all, how you can achieve it.

Health professionals are well aware that in order to achieve long-term weight loss, long-term changes in behavior must take place. This means changing eating habits, as well as including in your life some kind of exercise regimen, however gentle. As a profession we are all united on this issue—there is no debate. We know it is the truth. In spite of this, some unscrupulous companies, more interested in their bank balances than in our health, spend millions of dollars each year trying to convince us that the next "quick fix" is just around the corner, that their latest discovery really is the one that will rid us of those unwanted inches in record time.

This kind of marketing is very cruel.

The truth is, none of the quick-fix diets, including meal-replacement drinks and many other pills and potions, will work in the long term. (See Chapter 2 to find out why.) As soon as you return to your original way of eating, you repeat the process that made you overweight in the first place. In the meantime your body has become so bewildered that it is convinced it is going to be starved, and it learns to store fat more efficiently in order to conserve fuel.

Consumers are very vulnerable to advertisements and clever marketing strategies, and there is a desperate need to educate people so that they are not taken in by false claims.

I have written this book in order to dispel the myths. It just may be one of the most important books you will ever read, and I would encourage you to read all of it, from cover to cover. You will also find it very valuable to dip into from time to time, to remind yourself about certain things.

I wish you success. My goal is to help you achieve *your* goal, whatever that may be. Whether you want to lose sixty pounds or three pounds, this book will help you to achieve your goal. It will also help you to become fitter and healthier and allow you to get more out of life. That has to be good!

CHAPTER 1

Nutrition: The Bare Necessities

The Nutrients You Need and How to Get Them

How much do you really know about nutrition? My guess is that you probably already know that what you eat isn't ideal. Does this sound familiar?

> My diet is horrendous; I just don't have the time to eat properly. I often skip breakfast; there's too much of a rush. I have a light lunch, sometimes a bag of potato chips and a sandwich or just a piece of fruit. I have several cups of tea or coffee during the day, sometimes with a cookie, and my largest meal in the evening, which leaves me feeling full and bloated. I know I should make more of an effort, but I just can't.

How often have you felt a sense of frustration, or even failure, because you know you're not doing the best for your body? It's no wonder we turn to the quick-fix diets that promise magical results in short periods of time, only to find out that they don't work. In fact, we often end up in worse shape than before we started.

In this chapter I will outline the basic food groups: what they are and why we need them; how much we need to stay healthy; and how the energy nutrients are broken down to provide us with fuel. I will also give you tips to help you put all this into practice.

Why do we need nutritious food? The answer is quite simple—to provide our bodies with everything needed to function well, to give us the energy we need to go about daily life and to help prevent illness. It's not enough just to fill our bodies with bulk to get rid of hunger pangs; we need a balance of nutrients in order to achieve optimum health.

1

I believe the key to changing eating (and exercise) habits is learning to understand the body's needs. How often do we accept a new pill or powder just because the label says it's full of nourishment? If we can understand what our bodies need, how much is needed and why, it becomes much easier to see where we're going wrong and to do something about it.

So what is a diet? Going on a diet doesn't necessarily mean you are reducing the amount you eat in order to lose weight. Everyone is on a diet; it simply means what you eat. You shouldn't think of the recommendations in this book as something you should do, or as a diet you should go on, but, as I explained in the introduction, as reasons and ways to change—permanently. After all, if you can go on a diet, then you can also come off of it, and then you are back to square one.

Let's find out how much you do know about nutrition. With all the clever marketing that major food companies engage in, it is difficult to tell fact from fiction. Test your knowledge with these questions and see how you do:

1. Only fat, carbohydrates and protein give us energy.   true/false
2. Protein can be stored as fat.   true/false
3. Alcohol can be used to provide muscular energy.   true/false
4. Carbohydrates provide us with twice as many calories per gram as fat.   true/false
5. You have to eat meat to get adequate supplies of protein.   true/false
6. Protein is essential for hormone production.   true/false
7. There are approximately 21 essential amino acids (proteins).   true/false
8. A deficiency of even one of these amino acids can impair growth.   true/false
9. Potatoes contain protein.   true/false

10. A high-protein diet is potentially very dangerous.   true/false
11. Meat is a good source of zinc and vitamin B_{12}.   true/false
12. Fat vitamins are soluble in water.   true/false
13. Essential fatty acids may reduce your risk of heart disease.   true/false
14. Hydrogenated fats, found in margarine, contain trans fatty acids, which act in ways similar to saturated fats.   true/false
15. Cholesterol is a fatty substance found in animal fat.   true/false
16. The body can produce cholesterol whether or not you take it in through food.   true/false
17. Carbohydrates should make up the largest portion of the diet.   true/false
18. In order to burn fat, you must eat carbohydrates.   true/false
19. Dietary fiber cannot be broken down by the body.   true/false
20. A diet too high in fiber takes out essential vitamins and minerals.   true/false
21. Minerals are essential for blood clotting.   true/false
22. Vitamins can be manufactured by the body.   true/false

Here are the answers. Have a look and see how you did. The correct answer is in boldface:

1. Only fat, carbohydrates and protein give us energy.   **true**/false
2. Protein can be stored as fat.   **true**/false
3. Alcohol can be used to provide muscular energy. true/**false**
4. Carbohydrates provide us with twice as many calories per gram as fat.   true/**false**

5. You have to eat meat to get adequate supplies of protein.   true/**false**

6. Protein is essential for hormone production.   **true**/false

7. There are approximately 21 essential amino acids (proteins).   **true**/false

8. A deficiency of even one of these amino acids can impair growth.   **true**/false

9. Potatoes contain protein.   **true**/false

10. A high-protein diet is potentially very dangerous.   **true**/false

11. Meat is a good source of zinc and vitamin B_{12}.   **true**/false

12. Fat vitamins are soluble in water.   true/**false**

13. Essential fatty acids may reduce your risk of heart disease.   **true**/false

14. Hydrogenated fats, found in margarine, contain trans fatty acids, which act in ways similar to saturated fats.   **true**/false

15. Cholesterol is a fatty substance found in animal fat.   **true**/false

16. The body can produce cholesterol whether or not you take it in through food.   **true**/false

17. Carbohydrates should make up the largest portion of the diet.   **true**/false

18. In order to burn fat, you must eat carbohydrates.   **true**/false

19. Dietary fiber cannot be broken down by the body.   **true**/false

20. A diet too high in fiber takes out essential vitamins and minerals.   **true**/false

21. Minerals are essential for blood clotting.   **true**/false

22. Vitamins can be manufactured by the body.   true/**false**

How did you do? If you got some of them wrong, you will learn a lot of valuable information in this chapter that will help you to achieve your goal.

THE ESSENTIAL NUTRIENTS

The foods or nutrients we eat can be broken down into six groups:
- carbohydrates
- fat
- protein
- vitamins
- minerals
- water

The first three are our **energy nutrients**; in other words, they contain the fuel our bodies need to be able to function effectively. We burn calories, not only when we exercise but all the time, in order for our bodies to function and stay healthy. A calorie is simply a way of measuring the amount of energy we are using. One **calorie** represents the amount of heat energy it takes to raise the temperature of 1 gram of water by 1°C. A **kilocalorie** represents 1,000 calories. This is often written as Calorie, which means the same thing. All the calories from food come from carbohydrates, fat and protein, and this is why they are called the energy nutrients.

CARBOHYDRATES

Carbohydrates come essentially from plants; in other words, they are foods that are grown. They can be classified as foods that "have not been born." For example, pasta, rice, potatoes, vegetables and breads are all carbohydrates, and none of them has a mother. Plants capture the energy in sunlight and use it to produce glucose. When we eat plants, we are eating valuable sources of glucose, which our bodies can then break down and use as energy.

Carbohydrates can be classified into two groups: simple sugars and complex carbohydrates. On their own, simple sugars—such as glucose, fructose, lactose and sucrose—are **empty calories**. They have no significant nutritional value whatsoever; they just make things taste sweet. Unfortunately sugar is added to many foods during processing—you only need to look at the food labels on everyday items such as baked beans to find examples. More obvious food sources include:

• candy
• sugar
• honey

Complex carbohydrates are plant foods that contain stores of starch. They are more complex in their makeup, which consists of a combination of vitamins, minerals and fiber. Unlike simple sugars, they have a very high nutritional value and should make up the largest portion of our diet. Good sources include:

• fruit
• vegetables
• grains

Many people have misconceptions about the amount of carbohydrates they should eat if they are on weight-reducing diets. Carbohydrates are not fattening—fat is fattening! It is the fat (butter and oil, for example) that you put on the bread and potatoes that makes them fattening and not the carbohydrates themselves. However, if the total number of calories you consume in one day is higher than the number you burn, then you will gain weight as your body stores the excess as fat.

Recent research suggests that a diet high in carbohydrates and low in fat reduces the risk of developing some forms of cancer. This is because carbohydrates contain valuable nutrients that act as **antioxidants**. These antioxidants can deactivate harmful chemicals in the body, particularly if the carbohydrates are eaten fresh and raw. These harmful chemicals, known as **free radicals**, attack and injure vital cell structures. If you eat plenty of raw vegetables and some nuts and whole grains such as wheat, you will be getting an excellent supply of natural antioxidants. Good vegetable sources include:

- carrots
- spinach
- watercress
- asparagus
- broccoli
- green peppers
- brussels sprouts
- cauliflower
- red cabbage

Fruit sources of antioxidants include:

- peaches
- apricots
- oranges
- bananas
- apples
- strawberries

Antioxidants can help protect the body against many degenerative diseases, including heart disease.

Remember: Carbohydrates are a good source of fuel. They also provide valuable vitamins and minerals. If they are eaten in moderation, they will not make you fat. However, don't forget that too much of anything will be converted to and stored as body fat.

FAT

Fat is an excellent source of energy and performs many essential functions within the body. Certain vitamins can only be obtained from fat, and these are crucial for maintaining the nutritional balance we need. Fat holds your internal organs in place, makes up a large percentage of your brain and helps to connect your skin to your frame. It is, therefore, certainly not advisable to go on a fat-free diet.

You may have heard the term **essential fatty acids** (EFAs). These are simply fats that are essential for the body to maintain optimum health. Our bodies cannot manufacture these types of fat, so we must include them in our diets. The two EFAs are called omega-3 (alpha linolenic), which is found in oily fish, and omega-6 (cis linoleic), which is found in vegetable oils. Another fatty acid called arachidonic acid is semiessential. The body can make it, provided it has an adequate supply of other nutrients.

EFAs are vital for the health of your heart and circulatory system, as well as many other bodily functions. Not getting enough EFAs can lead to a deterioration in health and, ultimately, to death. (Deficiency symptoms are listed later.) EFAs are found in safflower, sunflower, corn, sesame, pumpkin and linseed oils. Other good food sources include green vegetables, tofu, fish (for example, salmon, mackerel, rainbow trout and sardines) and fish oils. Although all whole, fresh, unprocessed foods contain some EFAs, these EFAs go through many changes in the body, as the body has to break down and refine them into substances it can use. Many of us take in enough EFAs through the diet, but unfortunately, we also take in other foods that block the breakdown of the EFAs and prevent them from doing their valuable work. These foods include saturated fat, cholesterol, large amounts of alcohol and high levels of sugar. We should, therefore, not only think about how much fat we need but also look at the quality of the fat we are taking in. If you consider that every single cell in your body contains fat to support its membrane, you can see why the right quality is so important. If we don't take in enough of the good-quality fats, we can't use them to make our cells. Would you really like to be made from second-class materials?

If you're not getting enough EFAs, symptoms can include:
- eczema or dry skin
- hair loss
- liver or kidney degeneration
- excessive water loss
- susceptibility to infections
- failure to heal
- inflammatory conditions such as arthritis
- heart and circulatory problems
- deterioration of vision
- breakdown of nerve impulses within the muscles
- loss of motor skills (the ability to control muscular actions)

And so the list goes on. With many other major and minor conditions now being linked to a lack of EFAs, it is vital that we take in sufficient quantities through our diets and avoid foods that stop the body from utilizing these precious nutrients.

Having established the importance of EFAs, it is worth considering that most of us still eat far more dietary fat than we need and eat fat of poor quality; in other words, we eat too much of the bad stuff and not enough of the good stuff! We store this surplus as fat on our bodies. A high intake of the wrong kinds of fat drastically increases the likelihood of heart disease, heart attacks and many other serious illnesses.

The fat we eat is broken down into fatty acids, which will either be used to produce energy or be placed into storage in the fat cells. This stored fat is called **adipose tissue**. It is also sometimes called **cellulite**. The only time that fat comes out of fat cells is when it is burned as fuel. Fat will not be broken down by any cream or potion; it is a fuel, and any excess has to be burned.

The fat cell is constantly active, with fat going in and coming out all the time. If you maintain a balance between what you burn and what you consume, you won't get fatter. If the balance is tipped the wrong way, however, and you eat more than you burn, the fat cells will increase in size. (See Chapter 4 for facts about fat.)

Fat is either saturated (solid at room temperature) or unsaturated (liquid at room temperature). Most **saturated fats** are of animal origin (exceptions include palm and coconut oils) and contain high levels of cholesterol, which is another fatty substance present in animal fat. Cholesterol can clog up arteries and restrict blood flow if consumed in excess.

There are two types of cholesterol: good cholesterol (high-density lipoprotein, or HDL) and bad cholesterol (low-density lipoprotein, or LDL). It is the ratio between the two that is important. LDL carries cholesterol through the body and deposits excess amounts in the blood vessels. HDL mops up this excess and carries it back to the liver, where it can be broken down and excreted by the body (fiber helps this process). If the level of LDL is much higher than the level of HDL, then more and more cholesterol gets deposited in the blood vessels, which may ultimately lead to a blockage. Although every cell in the body has a need for cholesterol, the body is able to manufacture all it needs, provided its owner is eating a nutritionally balanced diet.

It is saturated fat that has been associated with heart disease. To restrict your intake of both saturated fat and cholesterol, reduce the amount of meat you eat and always choose lean cuts. Despite popular belief, beef is not exceptionally high in cholesterol and, in this respect, can be compared equally with chicken or fish. However, the total saturated fat content of beef

10

is relatively high, so it should be eaten in moderation.

Unsaturated fats are considered to be healthier than saturated fats. In fact, one particular unsaturated fat, olive oil, seems to be health-protective. A sprinkling of this oil on a salad or when cooking a stir-fry is a good way to get the essential vitamins provided by fat without the associated problems of saturated fats.

Fish—in particular, oily fish such as salmon, mackerel, tuna and sardines—is another good source of high-quality fat. The oils found in these fish can help prevent heart disease, since they block many harmful reactions that can cause blood to clot easily. The way you prepare your fish is also very important; don't fry it in butter or cover it in a creamy sauce. If you don't like fish, you may be tempted by the range of fish oil capsules currently on the market. Some of the higher quality brands, available in many health-food stores, are well worth taking. Always read the label and ask for advice before you buy— assistants in health-food stores are usually knowledgeable about the best kind of supplements. When you actually look at the amount of nutrients you are getting for your money, the more expensive brands often end up cheaper in the long run. More of the nutrients they contain can be absorbed by the body than can the nutrients in some of the cheaper alternatives.

It is worth remembering that fat is often hidden behind other names in menus and recipes. For example, cream is essentially fat, but somehow *fat of chicken soup* or *ice fat* doesn't sound quite so appetizing, does it? In reality, however, that is exactly what you would be eating. Just ask yourself, "Do I want to wear this chocolate bar more than I want to eat it?"

Remember: Some fat is essential, so select high-quality oils and keep to a minimum the amount of saturated fat you eat. The menus in this book have been carefully planned to give you the right balance of EFAs, while minimizing the amount of saturated fat.

PROTEIN

Proteins are often referred to as the building blocks of the body. This is because our muscles are made up of tiny strands of protein called **amino acids,** which give the body its basic shape and support. Since we are constantly breaking down these strands, they have to be continually replaced. Protein's other vital roles include maintaining healthy skin, hair and nails; producing hormones; aiding in sexual development; and sustaining healthy levels of red blood cells (which carry oxygen through the body). Although it is the second most plentiful substance in the body—after water—it is also the one energy nutrient we need the least of. As with fat, it's the quality of the protein we eat that determines our health. Provided we eat enough calories per day to satisfy our individual requirements, we will usually take in more than we actually need, so don't worry about the quantity.

Protein is broken down in the body into many different **amino acids.** The body is able to manufacture some of these itself, but there are eight essential amino acids that cannot be manufactured. A deficiency of even one of these eight can lead to problems with the production of protein structures.

Foods that are rich in protein do not always contain all the essential amino acids. If the food does contain all eight, it is termed **complete**; foods that are low in one or more are termed **incomplete.** Most meats and dairy products are complete protein foods, while most vegetables and fruits are incomplete. Ideally we should eat a mixture of animal and vegetable sources to ensure that we are getting the full complement. It is possible to get all the required amino acids from fruits and vegetables, but foods must be carefully selected. Vegetarians should take care to include beans or peas in at least two of their meals each day. They should also combine incomplete proteins

12

such as grains (cereals, pasta and breads) with milk or milk products (such as cheese and yogurt). Grains can be combined with legumes to achieve the same effect, and seeds can also be a good source of protein if combined with legumes. The proteins that can be obtained from vegetable sources are not as easily absorbed as those from meat sources. Vitamin C can aid this process, so vegetarians should always eat or drink foods rich in this vitamin with their meals. Good sources of vitamin C include oranges and orange juice.

Animal sources of protein include:
- meat
- meat products (such as pâté)
- fish
- fish products (such as paste)
- shellfish
- cheese (although you should watch the fat content)
- yogurt
- eggs
- milk

Vegetable sources of protein include:
- beans
- peas (including chickpeas)
- butter beans
- textured vegetable protein (TVP), often used as a filler in commercial products
- tofu and other soy products
- nuts and nut products
- bread
- potatoes
- cereals
- rice
- pasta (preferably a whole-wheat variety)

The body takes what protein it needs from these foods and breaks it down into amino acids, which it can then use. It is unable to store the rest as protein. (If you think about it, we don't have spare muscles tucked away, do we?) However, any leftover protein is stored as fat, along with everything else we consume in excess. (For information about the dangers of high-protein diets, see page 30.)

The Energy Nutrients—Picking the Right Combinations

A combination of all three energy nutrients is essential to maintain optimum health and to provide us with all the energy we need for everyday life. What we need most are carbohydrates, which should make up approximately 60 to 65 percent of the diet; next is fat, which should make up 25 to 30 percent maximum; and finally, protein, which should make up the remaining percentage.

If you think of your favorite meal (roast beef, gravy, roasted potatoes and vegetables, or lamb chops with peas and carrots, for example), you probably list the protein element first and foremost and plan your meal around that. Yet when you look at your plate, foods from the carbohydrate group—vegetables and rice, for example—should take up most of the room. The smallest portion should be from high-protein foods such as meat and fish. If this is what you see, then it is likely that you are achieving the correct balance between carbohydrates, fat and protein—well done! If most of the space on your plate is taken up by meat or fish, you definitely need to make some changes.

People rarely achieve the correct balance. Protein often makes up at least half of the meal. Because many protein sources such as meat and cheese are high in fat (often saturated), the balance is tipped the wrong way, and the majority of the meal is then made up of fat calories. This not only increases the size of your fat cells but also increases your risk of heart disease.

Food and Fiber

Dietary fiber comes from plant foods and is the only component of food that cannot be broken down by the intestines. This means that it comes out the same as it goes in. Fiber keeps the intestines mobile, which is very important. Some research has indicated that this may be cancer-preventive. By eating more fiber, you can also decrease your cholesterol level, which helps reduce the risk of heart disease. Good sources of fiber include:

• fruit
• vegetables
• legumes
• whole grains

Processed food loses much of its fiber content, often because the skin is removed from fruit and whole-wheat flour is milled into white flour. The brown varieties of bread and rice generally contain more fiber than their white counterparts.

If you are eating a wide variety of carbohydrates, you will automatically be getting enough fiber. Diets that are too high in fiber can be harmful, though, since food passes through the intestines before the digestive system has had time to extract all the nutrients. High-fiber diets require an increase in the amount of water consumed, since water will be absorbed into the fiber. If you do eat lots of fiber and don't drink enough water, you may develop stomach cramps.

VITAMINS

Vitamins are manufactured by plants, including fruits, vegetables and other foods from the carbohydrate group. The word "vitamin" comes from the Latin *vita*, for "life," and vitamins are indeed essential for life. They play an important role in the formation of red blood cells, bone building and many other functions of the body.

Vitamins are fat soluble or water soluble. **Fat-soluble vitamins**—A, D, E and K—are absorbed along with fat. The body usually has a store of these vitamins, and an excess can lead to the body becoming poisoned by them. **Water-soluble vitamins**—B complex and C—are more easily excreted by the body, via urine. Taking extreme quantities, however, can lead to dangerous side effects such as permanent liver damage.

Vitamin supplementation is big business these days. Powerful marketing strategies are used to sell us various combinations of pills and capsules, and many people have become convinced that in order to stay healthy they must supplement their food intake. In some cases, supplements are used instead of meals. I recently asked a friend of mine who regularly complains of a lack of energy what he'd had for breakfast. "I've had a multivitamin tablet and I'm full," he replied. There is a great danger here. No doubt about it—vitamin supplements can be very beneficial in cases of deficiency. When they are misused, however, they can cause more problems than they solve.

In an ideal world, there would be a plentiful supply of vitamins in the foods we eat. If you eat a wide variety of foods, you *should* automatically get all the nutrients you require. Much of our food is overprocessed, however, and so has lost a lot of its nutritional value before it reaches our saucepans. It then loses even more value during the cooking process, which means that there is very little left by the time we actually eat it. To minimize this loss, buy fresh produce whenever possible. Although it may be more expensive, you do get a lot more real food for your money.

If you decide that you do need to supplement, I recommend that you seek advice from a qualified nutritionist or dietitian before you buy. The way in which the body absorbs vitamins is very finely tuned; it requires a certain amount of each one. If one particular vitamin is taken in excess, the whole balance may be disrupted, and the body's ability to absorb other vitamins may

16

be impaired. Vegetarians are one group that does need to supplement because those who do not eat meat do not get the valuable B_{12} vitamin, which has many vital functions in the body. A deficiency of B_{12} can lead to anemia, so all vegetarians should take a multivitamin that includes B_{12}. The Recommended Dietary Allowance is a minimum of two micrograms a day.

If you discover you have a vitamin deficiency, the first thing you should do is examine your diet. It is likely that you are not eating something you should be eating. With the correct advice, this can be easily rectified. If you are sure that you are getting a well-balanced diet and still have symptoms of deficiency, seek advice.

MINERALS

Minerals are present in all living cells. They perform many important functions in the human body. Bones and teeth, for example, are made from living tissue combined with various minerals. Minerals are also essential for nerve transmission and many other metabolic functions. Some minerals such as calcium and phosphorus are required in large amounts; others such as iron and zinc are needed in smaller quantities. Eating a varied diet should ensure that you get all the minerals you need. This will depend, however, on the quality of the foods you eat.

One way of ensuring that you extract all the vitamins and minerals from your food is to avoid tea and coffee, particularly at mealtimes. Substances in these drinks can drastically reduce the body's ability to absorb nourishment, sometimes by as much as 50 percent. Try to avoid them for at least half an hour before and after your meal, or better still, don't have them at all. I have recently changed from tea to a caffeine-free instant drink made from roasted barley rye and chicory—it's delicious, and I don't miss tea one bit.

GOOD FOODS AND BAD FOODS

How do you tell the difference between a good food and a bad one? The answer is that there are no bad foods. I believe in everything in moderation. One chocolate chip cookie isn't going to do you any harm at all; it's the rest of the box of cookies that really does the damage! If you can eat one and be satisfied, great—lucky you! Most of us mere mortals cannot resist the temptation and just have to delve deeper into the package.

There are, of course, healthy foods and unhealthy foods, and if you educate your stomach and palate and get used to low-fat foods, even chocolate loses its appeal—I promise! Speaking as someone who used to devour two or three chocolate bars a day, I always considered myself lucky that I rarely gained weight; that is, until I got to 30, when, it seems, all my bad habits finally caught up with me. Suddenly I had to start watching what I ate, and chocolate was the first thing to go. It took me about four weeks to stop wanting a chocolate fix, but now I don't even miss it. I have strayed a couple of times, only to find that I still can't have just one chocolate on its own. So for me the only way to do it is to not have any at all. As for other so-called bad foods such as fast foods and french fries, if you have them only once in a while, you won't suddenly put inches on your thighs after just one meal. If you develop a taste for them and have them regularly, however, the inches will start to pile on.

NUTRITION—CHANGE WITHOUT PAIN

In order to make the necessary changes in your diet, you have to change the way you shop. After all, with the best intentions in the world, you can cook only the foods you buy. One factor that puts a lot of people off dieting is the thought of buying and preparing special foods and recipes. With this plan, however, you can eat a lot of the foods you are eating already; you simply change the quantities and the way in which the food is prepared. Don't expect to get everything right overnight. If you have to retrain your shopping habits and your palate, you need to give yourself time to adapt and experiment. If you force yourself to eat food you don't enjoy just because it's good for you, you won't stick to it. Remember: This isn't a diet that you go on then come off. These are lifestyle changes that really will improve the quality of your life. Food is one of the pleasures of life, and one person's pleasure is another's poison. So if you don't see menus that you like in this book, try to adapt the foods you already eat. Anyone can do it.

You could put all of your family on a highly nutritious low-fat diet, and they wouldn't even notice the difference.

TIPS FOR SUCCESS

✔ **Fill your shopping cart with carbohydrates.**

Buy More	Buy Less
cereals (check sugar content)	meat
bread	dairy products
pasta (egg-free and whole-wheat)	eggs (two per week)
rice	nuts
vegetables (all colors and textures)	sugar
fruit (all colors and textures)	
potatoes (don't fry them or cover them in butter)	
oily fish	

I used to curse the design of supermarkets. Everything always ended up balanced onto and crammed into the cart. However, the key to healthy shopping is learning how to work your way

19

through the supermarket so that you end up with low-fat, healthy items. Begin with the aisle where the vegetables are (usually the first aisle inside the door) and start filling the cart right there. Buy anything that looks good, especially organic produce if possible. Experiment with vegetables that you haven't tried before. Instead of having one vegetable on your plate with your meat and potatoes, have less meat and add two or three different vegetables—it's cheaper, too!

Next head to the aisle where you find rice and pasta for carbohydrates. Try different varieties—you have a wide range to choose from. With pasta and rice, however, try to stick to the unrefined egg-free, whole-wheat varieties whenever possible.

Then shop for cereals. By the time you finish this aisle, the cart should be two-thirds full, leaving space only for a small amount of meat. If you usually buy one pound of ground beef for a spaghetti sauce, buy half, plus an extra can of tomatoes, more mushrooms, onions, peppers and any other vegetables you like. You'll find that you can make exactly the same quantity, and no one will notice the difference. Now there should be just enough room in the cart for domestic items and no room at all for chocolate cookies.

✔ Always have breakfast.

Breakfast really is the most important meal of the day. Of all the possible mistakes you could make when planning your meals, missing breakfast is probably the worst. I am frequently told, "I don't have time" or "I'm not hungry." A recent comment was, "I don't like breakfast foods." Quite honestly these are all feeble excuses, so let's examine them one at a time.

Lack of time. Eating breakfast doesn't necessarily have to be the first thing you do every morning. If you have to leave early for work, take breakfast with you—yogurt, fruit or

20

some dried cereal in a plastic container, for example. Eat it mid-morning or when it is convenient. If you rise at six o'clock, you should eat before ten o'clock, if possible. The same applies if you have to get children to school—have breakfast after nine o'clock, when you get back. There are other things we have to do in the morning, whether we like it or not. How many of us would cancel the trip to the toilet to gain a few extra minutes to get ready? It's just as well that we don't have the choice—our bodily functions take over. Breakfast is also a necessary function.

Not being hungry. People who don't eat breakfast and have little or no lunch usually work up hefty appetites by the evening and consume more calories throughout the evening, often devouring cookies and other high-calorie foods. Such an eating pattern can reduce the morning appetite, so breakfast is missed again, and the cycle repeats itself. People think that if they don't eat all day, they can then eat as much as they like in the evening. Wrong. This is the time when our bodies burn fewer calories because we are less active, so we are more likely to store them as fat.

Dislike of breakfast foods. There are no set breakfast foods. Although we traditionally eat cereals and toast, there's no law that says we have to. I had this exchange one day while giving a talk on nutrition. One particular lady was adamant that she couldn't have breakfast because she didn't like it. I asked her to think of a favorite, easily prepared lunch, and she came up with a tuna salad sandwich. "Why not have that for breakfast? It sounds ideal—a low-fat, carbohydrate mixture. What's the problem?" I asked. "You just don't have tuna salad for breakfast," she said. Wrong. You can have whatever you like, whenever you like it. I have often

21

finished up the stew from the previous night with a slice of bread for breakfast—when I open the refrigerator, I just can't resist the smell. If my workload is particularly heavy and the children are waking me up at night, I often suffer from mouth ulcers, which make eating very painful. When this happens, I have a large bowl of rice pudding for breakfast, made with skim milk.

Don't get stuck in the breakfast rut: Vary the foods you have so that you enjoy breakfast as much as you do your evening meal. When you wake up, think of something low-fat that you'd like to eat and eat it.

People who do skip breakfast are likely to suffer from a lack of energy throughout the morning until they have something to eat. This leads to reduced performance and often irritability or headaches. Whether it happens at home while doing the housework or while working in the office, productivity levels will be low. The time you saved by not having breakfast is then lost tenfold because your body cannot function at its best. Breakfast kick-starts the metabolism for the day and is a must, whether you are trying to lose weight or not.

✔ Plan your meals.
If you have little or no breakfast, you are more likely to reach for that mid-morning snack, a bag of potato chips or coffee and a doughnut. A small lunch means hunger by the evening, and if you are too hungry, you'll eat the first thing you can lay your hands on—healthy or not. This is the time when the temptation to go down to a fast-food restaurant sets in and can be hard to resist.

One of the best gifts I have ever received was a slow cooker. When I'm working, it takes just five minutes in the morning— or the night before—to put some vegetables and meat into the pot with some water and a few spices. By the time I come home, the smell oozing from the kitchen is wonderful. In the time that it takes to boil some rice or potatoes, I have a satisfying, healthy dinner. I have also made spaghetti sauce, stews and curries in this way, and the extra cooking time always adds to the flavor and makes the meat really tender.

For lunch I often raid the refrigerator for cold vegetables, which I mix together with some low-fat mayonnaise and cold rice. I take this to eat at work when I'm hungry. This removes the temptation to buy sandwiches and other goodies from the bakery.

✔ **Satisfy yourself at each meal.**
This doesn't mean eat as much as you can; it means eat until you are reasonably full. Don't rush your food. The brain doesn't receive the message that the stomach is full for about 20 minutes after you've eaten, so wait a while after a meal. If you think you are still hungry after 20 minutes and the hunger pangs are still there, have a little more—if not, don't. It's a good idea to have an appetizer with your main meal, since your brain then starts to receive messages of fullness from the stomach when you are beginning your main course. Choose low-fat appetizers that take a while to eat, such as soup and bread or croutons with low-fat dips. Hopefully this will leave little or no room for that fattening dessert.

EATING OUT

How often have you started a diet with the best intentions, gone out for a meal a few days later and eaten all the foods you know you shouldn't have, felt like you'd blown the diet completely and then given up? Sound familiar? I hear this all the time from people who think that one lapse means that everything they've achieved over the past few days or weeks has gone out the window. While I don't recommend eating out often when you are trying to lose weight, the last thing I want is for you to feel like you can't go out. After all, that's the one thing that will make you crave a restaurant meal more than anything else.

There are, however, a few guidelines that you should observe. Go to a restaurant you know, where the chef doesn't mind making alterations to some of the dishes. I always ask for a low-fat sauce and no butter, for example. If you are going somewhere for the first time, make the reservation yourself and then ask if the chef can prepare you something low-fat in advance, including dessert. This is much better than asking when you get to the restaurant and finding out the chef doesn't have time.

Indian restaurants are probably the worst if you are trying to lose weight. Even so, it is possible to choose something low in fat and high in taste. Stick to tandoori dishes, particularly tandoori fish or chicken. Tikka dishes are also fine. Some sauces are yogurt-based rather than cream-based, and these are okay provided the meat isn't too fatty. You should ask for details, since each restaurant has its own variation on the same dish. Watch out for vegetable side dishes, which are often dripping in oil—ask the chef to cook one for you without oil. Vegetable curry can also be a good choice, with some plain boiled rice. If you have naan bread, make sure you ask for it without butter.

The dishes to avoid completely are the ones that contain creamy sauces, such as a korma, and also fried rice. They are literally loaded with fat calories—you may well carry the memory of your evening out for a very long time if you have one of these. For dessert have a sorbet—most Indian restaurants have a selection of different flavors. Not only is sorbet fat-free, but it will also clear your palate and refresh your mouth.

Chinese restaurants are probably second on the hit list, as they use large amounts of oil. I ask what type of oil they use

24

and have always been told vegetable oil because it's cheap and they use so much. You only have to look at an empty plate after you've eaten a Chinese meal to see the grease that's been left behind—you could write your name in it.

If you go to a Chinese restaurant where you know the food is cooked to order, ask the chef to cook yours with little or no fat. If the chef agrees to do this—and most will—you can enjoy a really nice meal without worrying too much. Chinese restaurants often offer steamed fish and may also steam some vegetables to go with it. This would be ideal with boiled rice. Again you could ask for this in advance when you make your reservation. Dishes to avoid are those containing red meat or duck and, of course, fried rice. Prawn crackers are like sponges that soak up the fat and should also always be avoided. For dessert, as with Indian restaurants, stick to a sorbet. You may find a lot of Chinese food to be very salty, which will probably make you drink more. Don't forget that too much wine or beer will also contribute to the total amount of calories you consume during the meal.

Italian restaurants usually offer both extremes. On the one hand, you'll probably find very rich foods in creamy sauces with lots of red meat, and on the other, you'll probably find a vegetable Bolognese sauce with some pasta and a salad (but watch out for the salad dressing). This second meal would be fine, as would be a small pizza, which can be cooked with little or no cheese at your request. Watch out, too, for olives—they are more than 90 percent fat! Although they are a very good source of quality fat, one or two should be sufficient—if you have them all over your salad or pizza, you will definitely be getting more than you need in one meal. You'll often find a larger selection of desserts than with the Indian or Chinese restaurants and should be able to get a delicious fresh fruit salad. (You can always take your own small container of low-fat ricotta cheese to pour over the fruit.)

Fast-food restaurants are a disaster if you are trying to lose weight; therefore, they should be avoided. Exceptions to this are certain pizza restaurants that now offer vegetable bolognese sauces to go with pasta and salads from the salad bar. (The dressings, however, may not be low in fat.) Some restaurants also offer delicious fat-free yogurt for dessert. If I want to take the children out for a meal, this is usually where we go.

If you do go to a burger restaurant, ask the employees which fat they use. Some chains may still use animal fat (saturated) to deep-fry french fries. If you find out this is the case when you ask, go to another restaurant instead. Better still, don't go to any. Don't be taken in by claims that the burgers come from 100 percent beef; remember that cows contain lots of unpleasant fatty parts that we definitely don't need to eat. The 100 percent beef promise doesn't mean you get only the good bits; the burger could be made from 100 percent of the garbage no one else wants.

CHAPTER 2

Busting the Body Myths

Diets Demystified and the Facts of Fat

There is so much misinformation about how to lose weight that it's not surprising people don't know which way to turn when a new product comes out. My heart sinks whenever I hear of new fads and gimmicks that are on the market, and I grieve for all the people taken in by false promises and clever marketing. I believe it is emotional blackmail: "Try this pill/potion/drink, and presto, no more fat."

Have you been taken in by quick-fix products? If you have had a weight problem for some time, then I'd be surprised if you have not. After all, faced with the choice of taking a pill or going on a diet to lose weight, don't we always want to take the easy option? Of course we do; it's human nature. Unfortunately, as I have already mentioned, none of these products actually works. They may even harm you and promote weight gain, which would of course make you a perfect customer for the next product that comes along.

I was recently speaking to a friend who is in her mid-30s and suffers from acne and blemishes. She said, "Janet, I never learn. I have tried every potion and lotion on the market, and yet each time a new one comes out I think, 'This is the one that's going to do it'—but it never does." Does this sound familiar? Is this how you feel about every miracle diet that comes along?

Let's look at a few of the myths that surround the diet industry. Here are some of the most common misconceptions.

✔ **Potatoes and pasta will make me fat.**

False. Both of these foods are carbohydrates and can make up a valuable portion of your diet. It's what you put on them that usually causes the problem. A baked potato smothered in butter will certainly be high in fat. If it is filled with raw vegetables in a low-fat dressing, however, it can make a nutritious low-fat meal or snack. Pasta also contains very little fat itself (provided you buy the durum-wheat variety and not the type that contains egg). A pasta salad provides lots of nutrients for a tasty meal. Both potatoes and pasta are quite slow to release carbohydrates. This means that they release glucose into our bloodstream gradually over a period of time, giving us a constant supply of energy. As a result of this, you won't feel full one minute and hungry an hour later. Of course, too much of anything—including carbohydrates—will cause you to gain weight. If the total amount of calories you consume is greater than the total amount you burn, the excess will be stored—as fat.

✔ **If I diet, I will lose fat from only one part of my body, so I can choose a diet specifically designed for my problem area.**

False. It is impossible to lose fat from one part of the body and nowhere else. As we explain later in this chapter, you lay down your fat cells at three stages of your life. Whether or not you fill them up depends on what you eat and if you exercise or not. This you can change, but *no* diet can empty fat only from certain cells and not from others. It's a physiological impossibility. You will lose fat from where you store it. So if you store fat on your stomach and you diet, you will lose it from this area.

✔ **If I don't eat all day and have just one meal in the evening, I will lose weight.**

False. In order to keep the metabolic rate elevated, we need to eat regular meals three or more times a day, depending on the amount we eat in one meal. When you eat only once in 24 hours, your body has to conserve fuel for long periods of time. To lose weight, however, you need to get rid of extra fuel quickly. The worst time to eat your largest meal is in the evening because you're moving more slowly and are less likely to burn off calories. It is much better to eat your main meal in the middle of the day, since this is the time when the metabolism is higher because you are on the move. There is another potential problem with eating only one meal per day: You are far more likely to eat more in one sitting than you would normally eat if you were having three meals per day. The bottom line is that if you eat more calories than you burn, you will store those extra calories as fat. Many people who eat one meal per day tend to pick and snack throughout the day on chocolate bars and cookies, since they are under the illusion that they are not eating much. All of these habits are more likely to increase your total caloric intake throughout the day one way or another, which means more fat.

✔ **Diet pills are a safe and effective way to lose weight.**
False. There are so many diet pills available without a prescription. Over-the-counter diet products can be on the shelves as long as they comply with labeling regulations and contain approved ingredients in approved amounts. However, many of these drugs act on the central nervous system and have potentially harmful and unpleasant side effects. A friend of mine was placed on a "metabolism booster" drug, which gave her hallucinations, violent headaches and insomnia. After a week on the drug, she looked and felt awful and was unable to continue taking it.

For those who do persevere, however, these drugs can be addictive. Appetite suppressants—or any other drugs associated with weight loss—should be taken only by clinically obese patients, when prescribed by a doctor. Even in these circumstances, it is still a very controversial area; a lot of researchers say that appetite suppressants shouldn't be used at all. There is a difference between foods that are advertised as helping you lose weight as part of a calorie-controlled diet (such as many diet drinks) and slimming products (such as those that promise to reduce your appetite). Remember: Even water will help you lose weight as part of a calorie-controlled diet.

✔ **If I eat just high-protein foods and limit my carbohydrate intake, I will lose weight.**

False. High-protein diets are, unfortunately, very popular at the moment. As you have learned from the nutrition section, however, we actually need less protein than any other nutrient. Not only do we not need excess protein, but if we take in higher amounts than necessary over a long period of time, we can damage our digestive systems. The protein we eat is broken down in the stomach by acids, while all other foods pass through the stomach relatively unchanged and are broken down in the intestines. Eating more protein means producing more acid, and if the delicate balance between acid and alkaline in the body is disrupted, digestive disorders may occur. Excess protein, like any other food eaten in excess, is also converted into fat and stored by the body.

✔ **I can get rid of excess fat by rubbing in cellulite creams.**

False. This is one of the biggest myths of all. Where is the fat supposed to go? I don't see it oozing out of the pores and running down legs. No, it stays exactly where it is. Of course, any kind of massage is good for circulation, but your fat cells will only release fat into the bloodstream to be burned when fuel is needed. The only way you can achieve this with a massage cream is if you jump up and down when applying the cream and continue to jump for 20 minutes or more, so that you stimulate your aerobic energy system into burning fat. A very expensive workout.

JUST WHAT ARE WE MADE OF?

We are all different. Each individual has a slightly different body composition, which can be divided into three elements: bone, muscle and fat. We often use the term **lean body mass**, or **LBM**, which means the combined weight of the bones and the muscles added together. Therefore, the remaining percentage would be classified as fat.

One of the most common reasons people give me for being overweight is, "I have heavy bones." Unfortunately for them, they have been misled. Bones are actually incredibly light—as strong as cast iron, but as light as pinewood. Fat and muscle—and not the size of our bones—determine our weight.

SO WHO'S OVERWEIGHT?

If you are overweight, it doesn't necessarily mean you are fat. Muscle tissue (which makes up most of our LBM) is an active tissue that burns calories in order to stay healthy. Even when at rest, muscles are still burning calories. Fat, on the other hand, does not need any calories; it just sits in its storage sites, stockpiling and doing nothing. Muscles are very heavy, much heavier than fat. This means that we can carry more weight in muscle and not be fat, even though the scales tell us we are heavier.

Imagine someone with a build similar to Arnold Schwarzenegger's. A very large percentage of his body is muscle, and he carries very little, if any, excess fat. If he used a traditional height/weight chart, however, it would probably tell him that he

31

is overweight. This is because such charts do not account for the fact that muscle is heavier than fat. Therefore, although according to the chart he may be overweight, he certainly isn't fat.

Similarly I have a very good friend, Carol, who is a fitness teacher. She is six feet two inches tall and weighs almost 180 pounds. This may sound a lot, but because her body has a large percentage of muscle and a relatively low percentage of fat, she is not fat. So again, although a height/weight chart may tell her she is overweight, she looks fantastic and turns heads wherever she goes.

As you can see from these examples, the scales do not always tell the whole story. What we need to look at is the body composition, not just the total weight.

EXERCISE IS EVERYTHING

If you don't exercise, your body composition will alter over the years, even if you don't change your eating habits at all. As I've already said, muscle is an active tissue that is designed to be used—to support the skeleton and to enable us to move. When we are using our muscles, we maintain the same LBM. If we stop using them or use them less, they will start to literally waste away. The individual muscle fibers become smaller and so require less fuel to function. This means, quite simply, that we then need to eat less.

Compare this to the engine in a car. Imagine a large luxury car with a very powerful engine. This engine would need a lot of fuel. You may get as few as 15 miles per gallon from this engine, so the tank needs to be very large. Let's say this car's gas tank holds 15 gallons. Now imagine a small hatchback with a much smaller, less powerful engine. This engine requires less gasoline, and you may get as many as 40 miles to the gallon out of the car. As a result, there's no need to put in as much gas, and the tank doesn't need to be as big. It may hold a maximum of 10 gallons, so if you tried to put in 15, it would overflow.

Now let's compare this to our muscles. Muscles that are constantly being used require lots of energy—in other words, food, for which they have large storage tanks within the muscle itself. These tanks are constantly being emptied and refilled. On the other hand, muscles that are not constantly used become smaller. They literally shrink, and their storage tanks shrink accordingly. So what happens if we try to put in the same amount of fuel that we put in our large muscles? It overflows. The body has a very effective way of mopping up this over-flow—it takes the leftover fuel and stores it as fat.

Take a 20-year-old woman with a total body weight of 120 pounds, for example:

Age	Total Weight	Fat Weight	LBM	% Fat
20	120 lbs	26 lbs	94 lbs	22

The amount of muscle will determine how much food the body needs in order to function efficiently. If we lose muscle through lack of exercise, we should reduce the amount of food we eat accordingly. If we don't, as we get older, we will be eating more than our bodies require and creating a surplus. This surplus will be stored as fat.

Now let's look at the same woman—who has not exer-cised—15 years later, to see what's happened to her body composition:

Age	Total Weight	Fat Weight	LBM	% Fat
35	125 lbs	38 lbs	87 lbs	30

Her total weight has increased by only five pounds. Over a 15-year period, most people would be quite happy with a weight increase of this amount. But take a look at her body composition. Because she hasn't exercised, she has lost a total of seven pounds of muscle tissue. As muscle requires on average 40 calories per pound per day, she should have reduced her total food intake by 280 calories (7 x 40). Since she has continued to eat the same amount that she did when she had an LBM of 94 pounds, she has overfilled the storage tanks of her muscles, and the excess has been stored as fat. This is an 8 percent increase in fat, which probably has had a dramatic effect on her appearance. (It would probably result in an increase of two dress sizes.)

PUTTING THE FAT AWAY

Fat is essential. We all need a certain amount of fat in order to protect our organs, and it also forms a vital part of many hormones, our brain and many other cells. We all have essential fat. There is, however, a marked difference between the way in which men and women store their fat.

Women were originally designed to be able to reproduce, so Mother Nature gave us extra storage sites for fat—on the breasts, hips and thighs—in order that it would be readily available to supply all the nutrients required to nourish a growing baby. Unfortunately Mother Nature was rather indiscriminate when dishing out these supplies; she didn't account for the fact that not all women choose to have children or for the fact that after we've had our families, we don't need these extra stores anymore. Many women struggle for years to get rid of a bulge that is, in fact, specifically designed to be there. They just don't understand why they can't get rid of it. The truth is, we can reduce these bulges quite drastically, but if that's where our fat cells are located, we can never eliminate them completely.

What you eat and whether or not you exercise are not the

only factors that determine how you look; genetics also plays a key role. It is generally accepted that we lay down or fill our fat cells during three stages in our lives. The first is while we are in the womb, and obviously we have no control over that because it is dependent on the genetic makeup we have been given by our parents. The second stage is the first 12 months of life. Again this is outside our individual control and dependent on what we are fed. The third and final stage, however, takes place during the "growth spurt" years, usually our early teens. This we do have more control over—but how many of us really thought that far ahead when we were spending our dinner money on a bag of chips and a can of soda? (Recent research has also shown that obese people can stimulate fat cells to multiply further.)

So when many of us reach adulthood unhappy about the way we look, we think we can change a pattern in just a few weeks or months that has taken years to develop. No, permanently changing body composition takes time, dedication and acceptance of what you are realistically able to achieve.

If, during all three stages, we have developed more fat cells than are necessary (remember that some fat is essential), it does not mean that they have to be filled with fat. Think of your fat cells as tiny sacks that take up almost no room at all when they are empty but lots of room when they are full. If you look at your mother and see that she stores most of her fat on her thighs, then the chances are that you will, too. However, you don't have to store as much. That will depend on what you eat and how much you exercise. Genetics determines where your fat cells are located—but *you* determine what and how much you put in them.

Men, on the other hand, don't need these extra storage sites and are given more muscle instead. On average, men store 10 percent less fat than women. But there's not all bad news for women. In fact, men are the ones who get the worse deal when it comes to the really important issue of health. Women store

more fat on their thighs and less around their abdominal cavi-
ties, which is where men tend to store most of their fat. Because
this area is much closer to the heart and other vital organs, fatty
deposits there are more likely to interfere with circulation. This
could explain the increased rate of heart attacks in men up to
the age of 50, as compared with the statistics for women of the
same age. Studies have shown that if men have waist measurements larger than their hip measurements, their risk of heart
disease is increased.

After menopause, however, women's fat deposition sites
change, since there is no longer a need for extra storage on the
thighs. Women then begin to store fat around the abdominal
area, the same as men. Along with this change comes the
increased risk of heart disease, which is much more common in
postmenopausal women. Postmenopausal women produce less
estrogen—which has a protective effect—so they become as at
risk as men.

There have been many theories about why women have
evolved the way they have. The body has an essential need for
the fuel that comes from the foods we eat—it's common sense.
In this day and age, most of us are fortunate enough to live in
an environment in which the food supply is never in question.
We always know that food is available. If we take a look back
at how we evolved, however, we see that it wasn't always
quite so simple.

Imagine a typical stone-age couple. Let's call them Mr. and
Mrs. Flintstone. Mr. Flintstone didn't go off to the office every
morning with his packed lunch, leaving Mrs. Flintstone at
home to look after the baby and do the baking. He went off,
club in hand, to catch and kill supper. Unfortunately for him,
however, he wasn't always successful. Some days he may have
come home with food and other days with nothing. Mr.
Flintstone was always the first in line for what dinner there
was; after all, if he wasn't fed, he wouldn't have the energy to

go out and catch the next day's supper. Children probably came next in line, with good old Mom bringing up the rear and getting whatever was left over. So life went on, with Dad using up his fuel chasing around after the next meal, and the children using up their fuel to grow and develop. Often there was very little left by the time the food finally got around to Mom.

As a result, Mom became very efficient at storing extra fuel, just in case she had to go without for a while or in case she became pregnant. That way she would have some fuel in order to nourish a growing baby. It was nature's way of ensuring the continuation of the species. Unfortunately for us, however, nature hasn't realized that some of us have a well-established food supply and therefore don't need these extra deposits.

Of course, this is only one of several theories, but if you are serious about wanting to change your body shape, you must first look around you at your family and your own history of diet and activity levels. Using this information you can then set yourself a *realistic* goal. (See Chapter 3.) The most important benefits you will achieve from this book—if you follow the recipes and the exercises—are the benefits to your health. You will have more energy; you will be stronger; your circulation will improve (which may improve your skin and your hair); and you will be able to really live life to the fullest, and probably live longer. You *will* also lose fat, and this will change how you look—but that is an added bonus. Think health first.

CHAPTER 3

Mind Over Matter

The Psychology of Dieting

Most of us diet because we want to change the way we look. For whatever reason, we have expectations that our lives would change if we could only lose weight.

Before you begin this program, I recommend that you sit down and ask yourself exactly what you want to achieve by losing weight. Prioritize your reasons. After all, you may find it very difficult to make some of the long-term changes that are going to be necessary to lose body fat. If you *are* going to make changes, you need a reason for doing so—a specific reason.

THE 28-DAY PLAN

I would encourage you to keep a small book or a few pages in your diary devoted to this plan. This will be *your* plan. In it you will individualize all the information I have given you, which will enable you to implement that information in order to achieve your goal.

BEFORE YOU START

You need to start your plan by listing all the things that are important in order for you to achieve your goal, such as shopping, cooking and exercise. You can start to evaluate in your mind things that are important. For example, making time to go shopping is important; it reduces the risk of being hungry with-

out any food in the house, which could then lead to the temptation to get takeout for supper. Exercise is important; it helps to
burn calories, not just while you are working out but also for
the rest of the day. Having ice cream, however, is definitely not
important to the success of your diet.

Now try to identify short-term and long-term goals. For
example, if you are saving for a new car, the long-term goal is a
car. That's all right, but it's a very vague goal; you need to be
more specific. Imagine your favorite car, one that you could
realistically afford if you saved, perhaps a green Jaguar. Each
time you are tempted to spend money, on a new outfit or a
night out, for example, you have to ask yourself what you want
more—the outfit, the meal or the car. Of course, it is possible to
have the occasional night out and still get the car; it will just
take you a little longer.

The first and most important step in setting your goal is to
be realistic. You have to be able to *achieve* whatever goals you
set for yourself, not just with regard to weight loss but also with
regard to any aspect of your life that you want to change. We
are all under intense media-generated pressure to conform to
certain images. Every time we open a magazine or a newspaper,
it seems we are faced with numerous images of the body beautiful. But how realistic is that image? It certainly isn't the norm—
it actually represents the minority.

Think for a moment of all of the people you see regularly, at
home or at work. Try to estimate how many people you are
thinking of. Now think how many of them have what you
would classify as a perfect body. Is it the majority or the minority? Of those with supposedly perfect bodies, how many have
achieved them by careful eating and regular exercise, and how
many were just born lucky?

We all inherit a genetic pattern from our parents. There's

nothing we can do about our basic makeup. In fact, approximately 70 percent of our body composition is predetermined. That leaves us 30 percent that we can manipulate, which *can* make a significant difference. As individuals, however, we also have limitations we must accept.

Unfortunately this is not recognized by the media. In virtually every aspect of life, we are constantly reminded that thin is in. How would Marilyn Monroe have coped if she were an actress today? I suspect she would have succumbed to the pressures and enlisted the help of a personal trainer and a chef. In adolescent girls particularly, the dissatisfaction with weight is so common that it has become the norm. Many young girls think of their bodies as ugly and despicable and constantly try to hide them, fearing others will view them with hostility and contempt if they are less than perfect. It makes no difference whether they are talented or intelligent—weight is their only concern. They feel that they will be judged by their size alone.

Self-acceptance is crucial—we are who we are. Before you start this program, sit down and write a list of things you like about yourself that have nothing to do with your body image. If you find this difficult, get a close friend to do it for you. Add this to your plan and keep it in a safe place. This will be very important for you during times of stress.

Next write a list of things that you *think* will change in your life when you achieve your target weight loss. Are these things realistic? Do you think people will like you more? Perhaps you think someone tall, dark and handsome will fall in love with you and carry you off into the sunset, or that you will get an instant promotion at work. You need to be realistic and acknowledge that such things are very unlikely to happen simply because you look more beautiful.

If wonderful things do start to happen to you once you've lost weight, it's far more likely to be because of changes in your personality, such as increased confidence and self-respect. You are more likely to take greater care of your appearance when you have a figure that you are happy with. Your attitude about various issues will change. You may find that you become a more positive person. Real friendship, however, will not change with the scales; it doesn't go up as your weight goes down.

Are you really ready to undertake this program? How serious are you about losing weight? When setting your goals, you must take into account your current situation. If you are currently in a stressful situation—like moving to a new house, changing jobs or having problems with relationships—this is probably not the best time for you to try to lose weight. You are less likely to succeed, and that in itself may lead to feelings of depression and frustration.

Overweight people are often described as jolly, but also as frequently suffering from feelings of inferiority and a deep need to be loved. While this is true of some overweight people, it is also true of others who have absolutely no need or desire to lose weight. It has been said that obesity (being 20 percent or more above the maximum desirable weight for each individual) is a person's way of handling a poor relationship with himself or herself. This view has now changed, and poor relationships are more often considered to be the result of the prejudice and discrimination often shown to individuals who are overweight, and not the result of the condition itself.

SETTING YOUR GOALS

What is a goal? It is an ultimate aim, a reason for trying. The first thing you need to do is to set yourself a goal for today. Write it down *now*. If it's not written down, it's not a goal—it's a dream. Next set yourself a goal for one week. (You don't have to start on a Monday—any day will do.) Set additional goals for one month, three months, six months and twelve months. Keep this list of goals somewhere safe, as part of your plan. As you achieve each one, cross it off.

The scales are not the only measure of progress. Go to your local practitioner and have your blood pressure and pulse rate checked before you start this program. These are important indicators of fitness, even though they are not visible. After three months, go back and have them checked again, and keep a record of your achievements in your plan. Go back again after six months, and again after one year, to see if you are maintaining your initial improvements. Write these dates in your diary now; as you see the dates creeping up, you'll be encouraged to keep up the good work. We all want to do well when we are having tests done, especially if they are going to measure our progress.

Once I went to a talk on motivation that was truly inspirational. The speaker, Mikki Williams, gave everyone in the room a rubber band, just like the ones with a locker number attached that you get at swimming pools. These bands were to represent our goals for the week. When we achieved our goals, we were to take the bands off. The results were surprisingly successful. In speaking to others who wore the bands, I found that most people actually did keep them on until they achieved their goals because they served as reminders that they had specific objectives for that week. Nothing had changed, their ability to *achieve* their goals certainly hadn't changed, but their *desire* to take off the bands did inspire them to accomplish their goals.

You could do the same thing. All you need is a thick elastic band. Tell yourself that the band is the reason you are eating less and exercising more. Don't take it off until you have achieved your daily goal each day for one week. And how often do you say, "I don't have time to exercise"? Try putting the band on and not removing it until you have exercised in some form or another at least twice that week. At the start of the following week, put it on and do the same thing again. You can use the band as often as you need to. Some people may need to wear it regularly, while others may find it useful to wear occasionally, particularly if they think they are going to be in a difficult situation. You may, for example, have several social functions to attend, and the thought of all those dessert trays is just too much to bear. Make a deal with yourself: "While I wear this band, not one cream puff will pass my lips." It will give you a reason for not having one. Try it; it's a surprisingly successful tactic.

Once you have established your goal of wanting to change your body composition and lose fat, there are several factors to consider before you set a target weight. First of all, what is the lightest weight you have ever maintained for 12 months? Second, are you prepared to make the changes necessary in order to lose the weight? You should take into account your current situation. If you are suffering from stress at home or at work, your chances of achieving success may be lessened, and you should take this into account. Be realistic about the changes you can make. They won't happen overnight, and there are several stages to actually changing behavior patterns.

CHANGE YOUR BEHAVIOR FOR GOOD

The first stage in changing behavior patterns is to contemplate change, but you will have already done that if you are reading this book. The next is to prepare, and that is what you are doing now as you read this. You are now acquiring knowledge that, if properly applied, will help you to achieve your goal, as well as knowledge about what types of exercise you should try and what foods you should eat. Then there is the third stage: action. This involves implementing the changes to your lifestyle, starting to exercise regularly and cooking with less fat, for example. Finally there is maintenance. Perhaps surprisingly this can often be the hardest stage. There are, however, several methods you can use to help you maintain your goal.

This strategic plan, from contemplation to maintenance, can be used in almost any situation. It, for example, reminds me of when I need to sort out my clothes closet. I spend a few weeks (sometimes months) thinking what a mess the closet is every time I go to get anything out. I promise myself that I *will* tidy it up. Then I try to plan a time when I will be able to do it, such as a quiet day or evening when the family is not around to interrupt me. When this time arrives, I take action. Everything comes out. I fill a bag for the next secondhand sale, organize what's left and put it away. Full of resolve, I determine not to let it get to be such a mess again, but maintaining my new method of "pants on the left, skirts on the right" is soon forgotten as the weeks and months go by.

This may seem like a strange analogy, but the principles are the same. Deciding to lose weight and to exercise is the easy part. Actually following the regimen and maintaining weight loss are harder.

One of the reasons for this difficulty is that we have to eat. It's not like giving up alcohol: You can't completely abstain from food because if you did you'd die. If you don't eat enough, you will deprive your body of essential nutrients it needs to be able to function properly. It is very important to accept that we need sufficient nutrients in order for our bodies to function— and that means food.

When you need to lose weight, it is likely that you will have to give up certain foods you like. You may find this quite difficult initially, until you experiment and replace them with lower-fat alternatives. But you can't just completely give up eating. This means that you have to learn to cope with the situations and foods that in the past have caused you to become overweight. But at least you are making these changes voluntarily. Imagine, for example, diabetic people who are suddenly told that they have to drastically alter their diets. It is much more of a shock to them because that is *enforced* change; at least you have consciously made your decision to change. Nevertheless, you will have to cope with various problems in order to achieve and maintain weight loss.

You need to develop an overall plan that will enable you to succeed. Examine how much time and effort will be involved in implementing your plan and how your plan will affect the people around you. How much time and effort is it going to take? Will it impose on other important areas of your life, such as family or work commitments? What will the emotional cost be? Is it going to affect your self-esteem? All these questions need to be addressed before you start.

KEEPING SCORE AND STAYING ON TRACK

You will also need to constantly reevaluate your plan and adapt it where necessary, depending on how successful you are at achieving your goals. Think of it as a cash-flow estimate for your business—one that examines expenditures and revenues to tell you whether or not the accounts will balance at the end of the day. If there is more going out than coming in, you know you need to alter certain elements of the plan and cut back on certain things in order to meet the payments. In the same way, if you are not losing weight, you will also need to cut back on certain things such as food and to increase others such as exercise. In this way, the plan should be constantly adapted to suit you and those around you. If it's not tailored to meet your individual needs, you are unlikely to stick to it.

If you are not reaching your targets despite eating the right foods (and not eating the wrong ones) and exercising regularly, you may need to reevaluate your original expectations. Every individual is different; I cannot give you a target that everyone will be able to reach. What I can give you are realistic guidelines. You should be able to lose between one-half and two pounds of body fat per week if you follow the menus and exercise programs. If you lose more than two pounds per week, it won't all be fat; most of the excess will be fluid. That's because the carbohydrates we eat help us to store water, so if we cut down on the amount of carbohydrates we eat, we are naturally going to lose some fluid. Once this new level has been established, the rate of loss will probably slow down to within the levels I have stated. You should take this information into account when evaluating your achievements on the scales.

YOU'RE NOT ALONE

When designing your plan, it is also important to ask the people around you for support. Consider how your actions are going to affect them. Perhaps someone else in the family will have to prepare the evening meal occasionally to give you time to attend an exercise class or to exercise at home. If you set the guidelines before you start, there needn't be any unpleasant surprises for anyone.

Equally important is to establish that your plan doesn't mean that everyone will be on hunger rations for the next few months. The changes you make when cooking don't have to affect the rest of the family. You will be able to eat many of the same foods as before, even though some will need to be prepared differently. It is, however, possible for the whole family to be put on a highly nutritious, low-fat diet and not even know it. Remember: A diet doesn't necessarily have to mean losing weight; a healthy diet can mean just eating healthier.

WHEN TEMPTATION STRIKES

Within your plan you should also have strategies for coping with temptation or relapses. It is asking a lot to expect yourself to be able to suddenly give up chocolate, cheese, ice cream or whatever your favorite high-fat foods are. Write down your favorite high-fat foods. Then write down exactly what it is you like about them. At first you'll probably say that you like everything about the foods. But you need to analyze your feelings and be specific. Is it the color? The texture? The taste? The feeling you get when you're eating it or the feeling you get when you've finished it? Next write down what you are usually doing when you eat these foods. This may vary from time to time, but you may be surprised to see a pattern forming.

Now ask yourself exactly what it is you are getting from these foods. Are you eating to satisfy feelings of hunger (in which case you've just been making the wrong choices), or is it to relieve boredom, perhaps while watching television, or do you eat to comfort yourself and relieve tension? Late-night snacks can become a habit; rather than trying to stop having them altogether (which will leave you feeling deprived), try having healthier options instead. Prepare some snacks before you feel hungry. Vegetables with a yogurt-based dip, for example, can be a very tasty low-fat alternative to chips and peanuts. I often make a large bowl of fresh fruit salad and dip into it whenever I am hungry. One of my favorite evening snacks is a bowl of cornflakes mixed with fresh fruit salad and low-fat milk. Cereal can also be a low-calorie, low-fat snack for any time of the day. Of course, if you are trying to lose weight, it is better not to have a late-night snack at all, but if you must have something, choose carefully.

"I only wanted one, but once I'd opened the bag I had to finish it. I couldn't help myself. I lost control." How familiar does this sound? What is this word "control," which we all seem to lack from time to time? The dictionary defines it as "the power to direct or determine." We do ultimately have the control, or power, to determine whether or not we will have one cookie or the whole box. Imagine your favorite high-fat food, perhaps a piece of chocolate cake. Picture yourself sitting in front of the cake, with a strong desire to eat it. If I told you that it was made with salt instead of flour or that even one bite would make you violently sick, would you still want to eat it? Probably not. But if you had *really* lost control, you would have to eat it, no matter what. The fact is, we don't lose control at all; we just choose not to exercise our control at a particular moment.

Visualizing yourself not eating foods that you will have to give up or at least cut down on can be a very good way of preparing yourself for facing unavoidable difficult situations— such as social gatherings, where you know tempting foods will be available. Visualize your host offering you a tempting selection of cheese and you saying, "No, thank you." Ponder this image several times, varying the situation and the food. It may sound a little strange, but positive imagery is very powerful. Think of world-class runners waiting for the start of the race ahead. Are they standing around chatting? Certainly not. They are busy concentrating, imagining running as fast as possible and breaking the tape, imagining and positively visualizing success. You, too, can imagine *your* success; it will help you believe you can do it.

HANDLING HIGH-RISK SITUATIONS

For real long-term success, you need to be able to identify high-risk situations—some predictable and some not—that will undoubtedly come along. You will have two choices, each leading to a very different outcome, both in the short term and the long term:

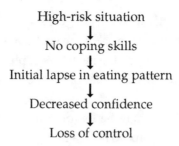

High-risk situation
↓
No coping skills
↓
Initial lapse in eating pattern
↓
Decreased confidence
↓
Loss of control

In this example, you don't have the skills to avoid the foods you know you should not be eating. You will, as I have mentioned, undoubtedly come across a wide range of circumstances in which you are tempted to deviate from your plan. If you do not know how to handle high-risk situations, you are likely to experience a short-term lapse, which may snowball into complete abandonment of your plan. This inevitably leads to decreased confidence and to eating more than you did before you went on the diet, perhaps in order to cheer yourself up, thereby making the problem worse than it was in the first place.

So what is coping? Coping is being able to identify high-risk situations and develop ways of dealing with those risks. First, and most important, you have to recognize what is high risk for you—this will vary according to your likes and dislikes. If possible, avoid the situation altogether, in order to prevent the problem from occurring again. This doesn't necessarily mean never going out; it just means planning ahead. For example, if you have been invited to a friend's house for a meal, you *must* tell your host that you are avoiding high-fat foods. You don't even have to use the word "diet." After all, if you are allergic to a certain food, I'm sure you don't hesitate to mention it, knowing that your host won't mind, as his or her aim is to prepare a meal that you are going to enjoy—not one that makes you sick after you've eaten it.

If you're eating out at a restaurant, you need to be aware of the kinds of food the restaurant serves *before* you go. If the restaurant offers only foods in rich, creamy (fatty) sauces, then try calling before you go to ask if the chef would prepare something for you that is not on the menu. Most places will be happy to do this—if your request cannot be accommodated, choose another restaurant. (See Chapter 1 for advice on eating out.)

Alternatively you may be tempted to go out for the meal and not say anything, just to have a night off. This means giving yourself permission to eat all the foods you have been trying so hard to avoid. If you do this once, you will find yourself doing it again and again, and your resolve and determination will decrease rapidly. Do you want to lose willpower or weight?

With a little bit of planning, you should be able to enjoy the same social patterns that you did before you started your weight-loss plan. If you start to decline invitations, you are depriving yourself of something that you previously enjoyed, and this can lead to feelings of resentment—not just for you but for partners and friends as well. In order to succeed with this plan, you must try to make the minimum number of changes to your normal social activities; otherwise you are unlikely to stick to it.

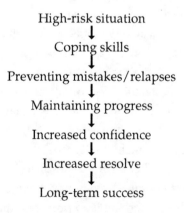

High-risk situation

↓

Coping skills

↓

Preventing mistakes/relapses

↓

Maintaining progress

↓

Increased confidence

↓

Increased resolve

↓

Long-term success

In this second example, you have developed the skills and tactics to enable you to handle high-risk situations. As you can see, the end result is very different from the first example. The situation was exactly the same; you just handled it differently at a very early stage. It may take you some time to develop the skills we talked about in this section, but they are crucial to long-term success.

It is also important to recognize that if you do lapse, it does not mean you have failed. If you lose one battle, you won't necessarily lose the war. However, it *will* weaken your defenses, so get straight back to the plan and determine not to do it again.

Exercise also plays a vital role in helping you stick to the plan. Many studies have shown that people who exercise have higher self-esteem and are less likely to suffer from stress. Because exercise is a positive habit (something that you do), it makes you feel better. Dieting, on the other hand, is associated with negative feelings and things that you *can't do*—"I can't eat cheese" or "I can't eat chocolate," for example. The good news is that the more you exercise, the less you focus on the negative aspects. The longer you stick to the plan, the more your physical image will change and your confidence will increase. And as low-fat, controlled eating and regular exercise become parts of your life, your improved shape and health will become parts of your life, too. And surely that is worth working for!

I hope this has given you some valuable information you will use to develop your own coping skills. Whenever you are faced with a difficult situation and are able to control it, write it down in your diary or in your plan in big bold letters—as a reminder that you can do it. On the other hand, if you have tried something that hasn't worked, make a mental note of it, and next time you are faced with a similar situation, try a different tactic. You will soon develop your own ways and means. Remember: It is impossible to lose control. Instead, you just choose not to exercise control in certain situations. It's up to you.

CHAPTER 4

Fat: The Vital Statistics

Everything You Need to Know About Fat

Most people think of fat as the excess we store on our bodies, but there is much more to it than that. The fat we store on our bodies isn't the same as the fat we eat, although some think that if they eat a cupcake it will go straight to their thighs. Well, it is true that it sometimes ends up there, but it is not a direct route.

THE FAT WE EAT

The fat we eat is made up of fatty acids that are bonded together to form long chains. Once these chains have been broken, the fatty acids can be digested. The difference between saturated and unsaturated fats is the way in which the fatty acids are held together in their chains. Saturated fats are held together by single bonds. They are usually of animal origin and are solid at room temperature. These are the fats that we should avoid since they are associated with an increased risk of heart disease and possibly cancer. Unsaturated fats are usually of vegetable origin and are held together by double bonds. They are liquid at room temperature and include both polyunsaturated and monounsaturated fats.

Polyunsaturated fats, found in corn, safflower, sunflower, cottonseed, soybean and walnut oils, were once thought to reduce cholesterol levels. However, researchers now believe that these oils decrease only the levels of high-density lipoprotein (HDL), the cholesterol that helps remove fat from the body, while levels of low-density lipoprotein (LDL) stay the same.

In addition, polyunsaturated fats often turn rancid when oxygen breaks down the bonds, causing harmful chain reactions that release free radicals. However, antioxidants—molecules that attach themselves to the free radicals—neutralize free radicals so that they become disabled and cannot cause any damage. Some vitamins and the minerals zinc and selenium are antioxidants. Many natural antioxidants can be found in green, leafy vegetables, which should therefore be eaten regularly.

Monounsaturated fats are also liquid at room temperature. These fats can be found in olive, canola and peanut oils. Unlike polyunsaturated fats, these are thought to drop levels of the harmful LDL cholesterol without reducing levels of the good HDL, improving the body's ability to transport excess fat to the liver for disposal. Monounsaturated fats are also thought to be less likely than polyunsaturated fats to oxidize—break down, turn rancid and release free radicals.

Scientists and chemists are able to change the structure of fat. Many of the spreads we buy contain hydrogenated fat—unsaturated fat that has been treated to make it become solid at room temperature, thereby enabling us to use it as a spread. This was supposed to have the health benefits of unsaturated fat with the spreading ability of saturated fat. However, hydrogenated vegetable oils contain trans fatty acids, which have been found to raise levels of LDL cholesterol as much as saturated fats raise them. As a result, experts say these oils should be treated as saturated fats are in your diet.

Hydrogenated fats are found in margarine, fried fast foods and processed foods, including packaged baked goods and potato chips. As far as what's better for you—margarine or butter—soft-spread margarine, with water or liquid vegetable oil listed as the first ingredient, is a good bet, especially if you are watching your cholesterol level. Olive or canola oil can be used for cooking.

PUTTING FAT TO WORK
FOR ENERGY

Fat is a great energy provider: Per gram, it gives us far more energy than carbohydrates. Our bodies are designed to make optimum use of this wonder fuel. A typical man can store about 150,000 calories in carbohydrates and a typical woman 164,000, which is enough to last approximately two days—but we have the ability to store billions of calories of potential energy in the form of fat. We also have a specialized system that enables us to store fat within the fat cells. If we had to store carbohydrates in the same way, we would all be huge, as every gram of carbohydrate also stores four grams of water. Our ability to move around would be severely limited. Thankfully nature has given us a far more practical solution—so the next time you're thinking how large your thighs look because they store fat, just consider how much larger they'd be if you had to store carbohydrates.

Unfortunately we cannot burn all this potential fat as energy without carbohydrates. Think, for example, of a marathon runner at the end of a race, totally exhausted because she has used up all her carbohydrate stores. Although she has billions of calories of fat energy left, she can't get to them—how frustrating! This means that you'll be disappointed if you go onto a very low calorie diet in the belief that you will be burning lots of fat from your reserve supplies. If you are not taking in regular supplies of carbohydrates, your body is unable to burn the fat, no matter how much or how little you have. Carbohydrate is the key that unlocks the door to the fat cell. You must eat properly if you want to lose fat. Very low calorie diets do not provide the amount of carbohydrates you need and also dramatically reduce the amount of water you store (remember the one-to-four ratio we mentioned before), which means that your total body weight will drop drastically even though you have lost little or no fat.

FROM YOUR FOOD TO YOUR FIGURE

So how does fat we eat become fat we store? The body is full of enzymes that help us to break down our food. Any enzyme responsible for breaking down fat and transporting it to the blood is called lipase. More specifically, the enzyme **lipoprotein lipase** is a long chemical arm that sits in the blood vessel and latches on to passing fat. It opens the door to the fat cell, throws the fat inside and then shuts the door. This enzyme can work very quickly or very slowly, according to how much practice it gets. Like all the body's systems, it can be trained to be more effective. If it is constantly bombarded with high levels of fat in the blood, it will work much harder and faster to take fat out of the blood and put it into the fat cells, filling them up and making the body fatter. Fatter people get fatter more easily and more quickly as this system becomes more efficient. The good news is, you can do something to change the rate and slow the work of lipoprotein lipase: Eat less fat over a long period of time. It is also possible to change taste preferences for fat in just 12 weeks; after that time the fatty foods you previously enjoyed can leave a very unpleasant taste in your mouth.

Insulin also stimulates fat storage. Insulin is a hormone—secreted by the pancreas—that monitors blood sugar levels. If the blood becomes bombarded with very high levels of sugar, insulin is released to escort fat from the blood to the tissues. If you eat foods that are high in sugar *and* high in fat, you are literally training your body to store fat. Ice cream, for example, is just sugar-coated fat. If you eat it, you eventually wear it. If you want to lose body fat, you need to avoid foods that are high in sugar, as well as those that are high in fat.

Fat cells are often called cellulite or adipose tissue. They are all fat cells, so don't be tricked by clever marketing. A fat cell is fat by any other name. Fat is constantly being sucked into the fat cells; it is a normal process—everyone is storing fat all the time. We tend to think of fat cells as savings accounts, where plenty goes in and very little comes out. In fact, our fat cells are constantly sucking in fat and spitting it out; they are active all the time. What determines their size is whether fat is coming in faster than it is going out, or vice versa. Either way, the system can be trained—and changed.

Saturated fats are stored very easily in fat cells. For example, the body finds it easier to store lard as body fat than it does olive oil (which contains monounsaturated fats). So if you eat 1,000 calories of each, although the energy potential is the same (1,000 calories), more of the lard is likely to end up in your fat cells than the oil. Overall, fat is more fattening gram per gram than carbohydrate because the body doesn't have to work very hard to convert it from dietary fat to body fat. Whatever foods you eat, a certain amount of energy provided by that food will be used to break down the food itself. In the case of carbohydrates, approximately 23 percent of the calories consumed are used up repackaging them for fat storage. In the case of fat, only 3 percent of the calories are used to make it suitable for fat storage—so there are more calories left to be stored.

If you eat a high-carbohydrate diet, you are more likely to consume roughly the amount of calories you need. If you eat a high-fat diet, you are almost certainly going to be consuming more calories than you need. It isn't difficult to overeat 800 calories in one meal if you choose creamy sauces and fatty meats, along with a high-fat dessert. On the other hand, it would be very difficult to overeat 800 calories of carrots. The reality is, of course, that so many readily available foods have a very high fat content. We have to make a conscious effort to read food labels—to see exactly what and how much we are eating—in order to keep our energy requirements roughly equal to our energy intake (what we eat). Many people who think they are eating a healthy diet are actually consuming far more fat than they need.

APPLES AND PEARS

Over recent years a lot of research has looked at how and where we store our body fat, particularly at the effects of storing it around the midsection of the body. Upper-body obesity is far more common in males than females, although it isn't totally gender specific. The fat cells in the abdominal area have a tendency to spit out their fat when they get too full. The fat then goes into the blood and circulates to the liver. To combat this, more insulin is produced, and it becomes a vicious circle. The fat cells that release the second largest amount of fat into the blood are those around the buttocks; the third largest amount comes from around the hips. This would seem to endorse the long-held belief that you lose fat from the top down.

LETTING GO OF FAT

Once the fat has been packaged into the fat cells, it may stay there for some time or be passed out fairly quickly to be used for energy. This will depend on two things: how much fat you are putting into the cells and how much you are taking out to be used for fuel. We have approximately 25 to 75 billion fat cells, all of which are potentially very active; fat is shuttling in and out all the time.

Fat cells have efficient systems for both storing and releasing fat. If both systems are working at approximately the same rate, you will maintain your current level of body fat. If one system is working faster than the other, you will be either losing or gaining fat. The rate at which fat passes in and out of the cell can vary throughout the day, but overall it will level out at a set rate, according to how you have trained the systems over a long period of time. This is called the **set point theory**. It means that the fat cells will protect their set rate of taking in and releasing fat—even if you change what you eat or the amount you exercise for a short period of time.

If you have been on a diet in the past and reached a plateau after a few weeks, it may be because your body is trying to protect its set point. However, if you continue to exercise, you will be able to change this set rate and get past the stumbling block in a matter of weeks. So don't lose heart—the plateau is just your body's way of adapting to a new set of circumstances. It is quite natural and very common.

The best way to cope with a plateau is to change something: what or how much you eat, for example, or the timing of your main meal. It may just mean eating smaller meals more often, or eating your main meal at lunchtime instead of in the evening. We don't have to stick rigidly to the regimen of three meals per day. I often "graze" all day, particularly in the summer when it's hot. As long as you are aware of the total amount of food you are eating and don't see it as a license to eat four or five large meals per day, it may be just what you need to kick-start your body into releasing fat. Because every individual is different, you will need to experiment a little, but always allow time for the changes to occur.

Many dieters experience a rebound effect about a month after beginning their programs, as their bodies try to defend their original set points. This is quite normal and should be treated in the same way as a plateau. Exercise also plays a key role. Perhaps you need to change the type of exercise you are doing or else exercise for longer. (See Chapter 6 for an exercise plan.) Remember: The key to breaking a plateau or a rebound is to introduce change.

If your rate of weight loss is very slow, it is likely that the enzyme responsible for releasing fat from the cell is working quite slowly. However, a steady rate of one pound per week fat loss is considered to be very healthy, and in the long term the weight is more likely to stay off. However slow your progress is, if you are releasing more fat from the cells than you are putting in, you are succeeding in your long-term goal—improving your health and your self-image.

Fat is released from the fat cells by an enzyme called **hormone sensitive lipase (HSL)**. This enzyme works in the reverse manner of lipoprotein lipase, which puts the fat into the cell. HSL sits at the edge of the cell and is stimulated by nerves to reach into the cell, scoop out some fat and put it into the blood, where it can be carried off to be burned as fuel. High insulin levels prevent HSL from functioning efficiently, so eating a high-sugar meal not only enhances your ability to store fat quickly and efficiently but also locks fat in the cell so that it can't get out. This is a very good reason for not eating ice cream or any other sugar and fat combination. On the other hand, if you want to put fat in your fat cells, that's the best way to do it.

Fat is stored all over the body. We always have fat in the blood readily available for use, and we can also store large amounts within the muscles. To improve body composition, however, we need to stimulate the release of fat from the fat cells into the blood where it can be used up. Exercise is one of the best ways to improve body composition because the burning of fat takes place in the muscle. In fact, the only place where you can burn fat is in the muscle.

By exercising regularly, you can train your body to metabolize more fat more quickly, not just when you are exercising *but all the time*. It's this process that will really accelerate fat loss. We actually burn relatively little fat while we are working out, but because we increase the ratio of lean body tissue to fat mass on the body, we increase the amount of fat and calories we burn every day in just staying alive. If you exercise regularly, you can burn more fat even when you are asleep. That has to be good news. The cruel truth is, if you don't change your habits and you are fat, you will just get fatter. This will have serious implications for your health and affect how you feel about yourself and the way you look.

It should be noted at this point that you must be careful about restricting a child's intake of fat. This is because fat is vital in the creation of the sheaths that surround and protect our nerves as we grow and develop. Children up to the age of five should, therefore, have whole milk. What you can do, however, is change the quality of the fat they are getting by restricting saturated fats and encouraging them to eat oily fish and unsaturated fats. Cooking with extra-virgin olive oil is much healthier, for example. Rolls with sesame seeds—preferably served without a greasy burger in the middle—are also an excellent source of natural oils.

CHAPTER 5

Exercise: Why Bother?

What's in It for You?

Unfortunately most people don't bother with exercise. A 1991 Centers for Disease Control and Prevention (CDC) study found that some 58 percent of adults report getting little or no leisure-time exercise, and that 24 percent or more are completely sedentary. Only 22 percent of adults are active enough to meet the recommendations for exercise set by the CDC and the American College of Sports Medicine—30 minutes or more of light or moderate physical activity on most or all days of the week.

Yet exercise is one of the most important factors that determine your health. Studies show that 300,000 deaths a year can be attributed to poor eating habits and lack of exercise. And yet physical activity can help to decrease the risk of heart disease, high blood pressure, type-II diabetes, arthritis, osteoporosis and even some forms of cancer.

HOW FIT IS FIT?

Some time ago, I toured the country presenting a talk called "Why Exercise?" to groups consisting mostly of women. I began each talk by discussing the definition of fitness, and the different groups came up with their own definitions of what it actually means. Overall each group had very similar ideas. These included:

- Being able to get through the day without feeling shattered

- Having enough energy to do the housework and play with the children
- Being able to walk to work and use the stairs instead of the elevator
- Having enough energy to walk the dog without getting out of breath

All of these are very accurate definitions of fitness and describe what fitness means to each individual. What would your definition of fitness be?

Having discussed the merits of being fit, I then asked the women (and some men) to write down the name of someone they could think of who was fit. Their suggestions included Arnold Schwarzenegger, Michael Jordan, Jackie Joyner-Kersee and many other similar figures. These are all elite athletes, people who, through very intensive training, have become the best in the world. I then asked them to look again at their original definitions of fitness, and together we went through the list and asked the questions: "Were these athletes fit enough to get through the day without feeling shattered?" "Could they walk the dog without getting out of breath?" The answer to both these questions was clearly "yes," but most important, did these athletes actually need to be as fit as they were in order to do these everyday things? The answer was, of course, "no."

Many people today seem to have the preconceived idea that fitness is something unachievable. When I talk about fitness, I am talking about the following: a body that is healthy enough to be able to withstand disease; a body that can recover quickly from minor illness; a body that allows its owner freedom to complete everyday tasks without the restrictions of breathlessness and discomfort.

The human body is nothing short of a miracle. I have been designing workouts and studying nutrition for more than 15 years, and yet it still astounds me that the body uses so many interrelated and complicated systems in order to function. In addition to this, I have seen people literally change their lives and their health—not to mention their shapes—just by training their bodies and teaching them to improve their efficiency. There is no piece of machinery in the world that has this ability to improve itself by training, but the human body can. The secret is quite simple—challenge your body to work slightly harder than it does already.

How many of us could recite our 13 times table if asked? I certainly couldn't because I have only been programmed to recite my tables up to 12. Your body has the same limitations—it will function only according to the demands you place on it and no more. If you don't exercise regularly and don't challenge your heart and muscles, they will become smaller and weaker because your body thinks they are not needed. All you need to do to reverse this process is to start to place gentle demands on your body's systems. If you do this regularly, your body will get stronger and improve itself in order to adapt to the new demands. The heart will get stronger and pump more blood, and the muscle fibers will get stronger to give you more strength. In fact, muscle fibers can even get longer to allow you more flexibility.

The good news is that you don't have to work very hard for these miraculous changes to occur. You will, in fact, reap the most benefit in the first few weeks of training. Someone who has never exercised can improve fitness levels by a staggering 25 to 35 percent in the first few weeks. You will start to feel fitter because you will be teaching your body to use more of the oxygen you are breathing to help provide you with energy.

FINDING YOUR WAY TO EXERCISE

With what do you associate the word "exercise"? Most people who don't exercise associate it with pain or discomfort. For some the mere mention of the word sends shivers down the spine, conjuring up visions of cross-country runs and high school gym classes. I can remember several less than pleasant exercise experiences at school: playing hockey with sticks that left me with bruises up to my knees; defending a goal against an attacker who was so much taller than I that she almost stepped on me as she went past; spending an hour or more serving tennis balls into the net, driving my opponent into a rage.

Despite all this, however, I was very fortunate in that even though I hated all the outdoor sports, once I was in the warm and cozy gymnasium—with soft crash mats and lots of ropes and poles to swing around on—I loved it. The result of finding an activity I really enjoyed was that I started to do more of it and, before long, was training regularly and entering competitions. The moral of this story is quite obvious—you have to find some kind of activity that you enjoy, or you won't stick to it. You need to choose a form of exercise that you can do without dread. If you find something you are good at, you will want to do it more—it's human nature. Your motivation will also increase after a month or so as you start to see and feel the benefits.

You may find that you prefer to exercise with someone else or in a group setting. Look in your local paper for details of fitness classes in your area. It doesn't have to be aerobics; there are lots of different types of classes. It will not necessarily matter which one you choose—all exercise has a very important part to play if you are serious about losing weight.

If you are going to go to an organized class, make sure that the instructor is qualified. In the United States, the Aerobics and Fitness Association of America and the American Council on Exercise award certification to qualified instructors who have completed workshops on teaching techniques, anatomy, physiology and exercise safety and who have completed a practical and written exam. Don't be afraid to ask your instructors about their qualifications—if they are certified, they will have worked so hard to earn it that they will be only too happy to tell you. Unfortunately not all teachers who qualify continue to maintain such high standards once they have passed the exam. Do you drive your car in the same way you did for your driving test? Probably not.

The fitness industry is constantly changing. We are learning more about the body all the time, and as we learn more about how the body adapts to exercise, we are able to design safer training programs. It is vital, therefore, that instructors are up-to-date on the latest information. Good instructors will regularly attend seminars and training courses to make sure that the information they are giving is correct. Here are some questions you should consider when choosing fitness instructors:

- Did they ask you to complete a health questionnaire before beginning the class?
- Do they regularly check that everyone is all right—no recent injuries or illnesses, for example?
- Does the class always begin with a gentle warm-up? (You should never feel breathless in the warm-up.)
- Do they constantly remind you about good technique and posture?
- Do they give good demonstrations of what they want you to do?
- Do they move around to make sure that everyone is doing the exercise correctly, or are they too busy having a workout themselves?
- Do they help or correct participants who are not in the right position?
- Can you hear the instructions clearly above the music?

- Do they face the class and really look at individuals, as opposed to facing the mirror and watching themselves?
- Do they always offer alternatives for people of varying fitness levels?
- Do you feel that it's your workout or theirs?
- Do they make themselves available for questions before or after the class, or are they always talking about themselves and what they can do?

These are just a few of the qualities to look for when choosing instructors. Don't be afraid to be choosy; after all, you are putting your body in their hands. If you make a bad choice, you could end up getting injured.

Of course, you don't have to go to an exercise class to have a good workout. There are lots of other alternatives, and what is offered in a class may not suit everyone. For example, some people would benefit from activity levels that are not strenuous or not particularly long in duration. It is certainly not compulsory to experience the "high" sensation that some people get from exercising to the point of near exhaustion. It's important to remember that *most* people don't actually like the feeling of being hot and sweaty with aching limbs. What they do like, however, is the feeling of satisfaction and well-being they experience after they have exercised, a feeling that can last for several hours. You'll find a list of alternatives to classes in the following chapter—choose whatever's right for you.

REAPING THE REWARDS

When I was teaching fitness classes three nights per week, I often used to sit on the sofa half an hour before I was due to leave and wish that I didn't have to go. I used to think, "I can't be bothered." Does that sound familiar? How many times do you make that excuse? Or perhaps you say, "I'm too tired" or "I haven't got time." I am now thankful that I did go since I have managed to stay healthy and in good shape as a result. You would be amazed at how many people say to me, "You're so lucky to have a figure like that," when, in fact, luck has little to do with it. It's true that I have never been drastically over-weight, but that is because I have always watched what I've eaten and have exercised regularly. I am as predisposed as most people to gaining weight, particularly since I have grown older. However, it's not just my figure—my skin and hair really suffer if I eat greasy foods and don't work out. I feel grumpy and lethargic and lose the motivation to want to exercise, which, of course, makes the situation worse.

Exercise can help us in so many ways. Weight loss is just one benefit, although it is perhaps the most visible. There are, however, many psychological benefits, including being better able to cope with stress; being less likely to suffer from depres-sion; being able to recover more quickly from illness—and so the list goes on.

The beauty of exercise is that the benefits are so long lasting. If you work out for an hour in the morning, the benefits you gener-ate will keep on working for hours afterward. Your metabolic rate will increase, which means you will burn more calories—including fat. Your heart and other muscles will adapt to the new demands and will make themselves stronger—this also requires more calories. Your circulation and digestive system will also benefit, and all this will happen while you go about your daily tasks. It reminds me of a commercial on television for a mouth-wash. In the first shot, you see a man getting ready for work, brushing his teeth and using the mouthwash. A few minutes later, after another commercial, up pops the same man suppos-edly later in the day at work. He smiles and says, "It's still work-ing." A few minutes later, after yet another ad, the same man appears in the evening scene with the same comment, "It's still working." The benefits are still being achieved hours after the event has taken place—it's exactly the same with exercise.

It's not just the energy cost of the exercise that is important— that is, how many calories you burn up while actually working out—it's how many calories you need to burn just to stay alive. If you are overweight, there is visible evidence that you are eating more than you need. If you exercise regularly, however, that daily requirement—the number of calories you need to stay alive and healthy—will increase as you replace lost muscle tissue, and you really will burn more calories 24 hours per day, even while you sleep. That's one kind of exercise we all have to find time for.

Good health and the prevention of disease are basic human needs. We invest huge sums of money trying to buy health, when we actually have most of the answers completely free of charge. With regular exercise you can extend your life span by several years, not to mention drastically improve your quality of life. Think ahead for a moment. If you cannot stand up from a chair unaided, then you cannot get off the toilet unaided. This means that your chances of living at home and not being institu- tionalized when you get older are slim because your muscles and heart will have weakened so much due to inactivity that you will no longer be able to look after yourself. Exercise is not just about losing weight; it is a free prescription for a healthy body.

IT'S NEVER TOO LATE

People often tell me that they are too old to exercise, but that is simply not true. Provided you are in good general health, there is no reason whatsoever that you cannot begin a gentle exercise program and reap the same benefits as someone younger. There is little or no difference between the improve- ments gained by elderly people starting exercise programs and those achieved by people in their 20s.

In a recent study, scientific researchers wanted to test this theory. They went to their local residential care center and asked for some volunteers to start an exercise program. They were met initially with cries of horror from the staff, but once they'd persuaded them that it was all perfectly safe and that the participants would be very well supervised, they did manage to get a few residents to join in. These residents felt that they had nothing better to do since they were only sitting around anyway. The program began very gently with some mobility work in a chair and, over the course of a few months, progressed to include some strength work to try to regain some of the muscle tissue lost due to years of inactivity. At the same time, similar exercise programs were carried out with college students. The workouts were adapted to their increased level of fitness, and both groups worked at approximately 80 percent of their maximum potential.

When the results were compared at the end of the program, it was noted that the residents had dramatically improved their quality of life. They were more active during the day; they were more likely to play table tennis and go for walks rather than just sit around all day; and their medication requirements had gone down—in some cases, quite drastically. In addition to this, the results of the original test—which was to see whether or not they could gain the same improvements in muscle tissue as the younger students—showed clearly that they could. The replacement of lost muscle tissue was far more significant to the residents than it was to the younger group because it literally changed their lives. When the researchers completed their study, they were persuaded to stay and design a much larger program for the other residents, who had seen the changes in those who had taken part and wanted the same benefits themselves. The oldest resident who took part in the study was in his 90s.

THE RIGHT PROGRAM FOR YOU

So what is the best form of exercise for you? The answer is very simple—it's the form of exercise that you enjoy doing and that fits in best with your daily routine. If it doesn't fit into your lifestyle without any major changes, you will not stick to it.

In order to work out the best exercise program for you, you need to decide exactly what you want to achieve by exercising—weight loss, for example. Different types of exercise have different effects on the body, and the exercise programs in this book have been specifically designed to help you lose weight. I believe you are more likely to stick to an exercise program if you understand exactly what is going on inside your body while you are working out. So let's take a look at the body's energy systems.

It may surprise you to learn that we have several ways of producing the energy required to make our muscles contract and that not all of these ways burn fat. The body is able to utilize different foods—such as fat, carbohydrates and protein—in different ways in order to provide us with energy. These foods are the energy nutrients. (See Chapter 1.) Just as we have a choice between which fuels we use in our homes, the body has two main energy systems to choose from. Which one we use is determined by the following: how many muscles are working; how hard they are working; how fast they are working; and what foods are available to provide the fuel.

THE AEROBIC ENERGY SYSTEM

This is by far the most efficient of the two systems. **Aerobic** means that the body is using oxygen to help it break down the food molecules that are being used to provide energy. The foods required for this are carbohydrates (which are broken down into glycogen, or blood sugar) and fats (which are broken down into fatty acids). Together these go through a series of chemical changes within the muscle, giving it the power to contract.

Unfortunately we cannot burn fat without glycogen. One of the reasons so many people fail with low-calorie diets is that they are not eating enough carbohydrates to provide the glycogen necessary to burn fat. They may lose body weight, but as explained in Chapter 2, although they end up weighing less, they have a higher percentage of fat on their bodies and so look very flabby. As soon as they resume a normal eating pattern, they regain all their lost weight and more.

The aerobic energy system is very similar to gas central heating—it takes a long time to get going, but once it does, it is extremely cost effective and the output is very good. It gives us lots of energy for long periods of time, provided we are not working too hard. It is entirely dependent on the efficiency of the cardiovascular system (the heart and blood vessels) in pumping oxygen through the body and into the cells (inside the working muscles), which break down the fat and glycogen. Examples of the types of activity that use aerobic energy include walking, swimming, jogging and cycling.

Each individual has a different aerobic capability based on the efficiency of the heart and lungs. As soon as the level of the activity becomes too high, the body switches to the anaerobic energy system.

THE ANAEROBIC ENERGY SYSTEM

This second energy system comes into effect when the heart cannot pump oxygen around the body quickly enough. It breaks down glycogen but not fat, and it does so without the use of oxygen. We use this system when the need for energy is greater and more immediate. Examples of anaerobic activities include racquetball, sprinting, high or long jump and other short-term, power-based events.

If you came home to a cold house, an electric fan heater would give you more heat more quickly than gas central heating. The anaerobic energy system also gives us more power more quickly. However, the disadvantage is that we cannot keep going at a high level of intensity for very long. The reason for this is that we can store only limited amounts of glucose in the muscle (muscle glycogen), and when this runs out, we have to wait for the liver to process some more and to deliver it to the muscle. On the other hand, with the aerobic energy system the supply of glycogen lasts much longer because fat is providing most of the fuel, and glycogen stores are spared.

HOW HARD SHOULD YOU WORK?

One of the biggest areas of controversy concerns how hard you should work in order to maximize the amount of fat you burn while you are working out. The truth is that whatever form of exercise you do, you will be helping your body to burn fat, not only while you are exercising but all the time. One school of thought is that if you work too hard, you *won't* burn fat. This is based on the principle that because it takes a long time for the fat to be taken out of the fat cells, into the bloodstream, into the muscle and then finally broken down, you need to exercise for quite a long time in order to stimulate this process. In other words, by the time the fat has been taken to the muscle, you will have already finished exercising. There is a lot of scientific evidence to support this, and in principle it is true.

To maximize the amount of fat you burn while you are working out, you should aim to keep going for longer to give your fat cells more time to release their fat. You should also remember that if you do this regularly, you will be training your fat cells to release fat into the bloodstream to be used as fuel. (See Chapter 4.) In order to do this, you will need to keep the level of exercise fairly low to moderate—after all, Olympic gold medalist Carl Lewis could not run as fast over 1,500 meters as he does over 100 meters. In general terms, you should feel breathless but not exhausted. (See the activity level scale on pages 79–80.)

There are several ways in which you can estimate how hard you are working in order to see whether or not you are burning fat. The first is to take your pulse rate while you are at the hardest point of the exercise. The problem with this, however, is that if you are moving around (jogging or swimming, for example), it is almost impossible to take your pulse accurately. You will also need to calculate in advance what your maximum pulse rate should be. You can do this by using a simple system of subtraction. Start with 220 and deduct your age. As an example, for a 30-year-old the equation would be as follows:

$$220 - 30 = 190$$

So 190 beats per minute would be the **maximum training heart rate**. In other words, this is the maximum speed that person's heart can beat at, so we will call this 100 percent:

$$220 - 30 = 190 = 100\%$$

Obviously you don't want to work at 100 percent. Research has shown that when we work at approximately 65 percent we burn the most fat. Sixty-five percent of 190 is 123. Therefore, if a 30-year-old reaches a level where the heart is beating 123 times per minute, he or she is likely to be in the "fat-burning zone":

$$220 - 30 = 190$$
$$65\% \text{ of } 190 = 123$$

Isn't that good news? Instead of going flat out on an exercise bike or a stair climber and feeling exhausted after five minutes, what you need to do is to pedal away at a level that is comfortable and sustainable. Remember: It takes longer to start burning fat than just glycogen alone, so start gently and gradually increase the time you spend on the activity, until you can work at a comfortable level for 20 or 30 minutes. Rest assured, you *will* be burning fat. You will also be improving your cardiovascular system and reducing your risk of heart disease.

The second school of thought is completely different, but also correct. It is based on the total amount of calories burned during exercise. Having established that you burn a higher percentage of calories from fat if the level is low to moderate, we now need to look at the total number of calories burned overall during low- versus high-intensity exercise. The following table shows the difference between the total calories burned during walking and running:

	Walking	*Running*
Distance	4 miles	6 miles
Speed	4 mph	6 mph
Time	60 minutes	60 minutes
Total Calories	270	680
% Fat Calories	60	40
Total Fat Calories	162	272

By looking at these figures, we can see that we do burn a higher percentage of fat calories when the activity is low to moderate, and that is good news for those of us who don't like to work too hard. However, we must also look at the *total number of fat calories burned* in order to see the whole picture. Although we burn 60 percent of calories from fat when we are walking, as opposed to only 40 percent when running, the total number of fat calories burned is higher when running because the overall total is so much greater (40 percent of 680 is more than 60 percent of 270). This should not be taken too literally, however, as the figures shown are based on running for 60 minutes, which is unachievable for most of us. I certainly could not run for 60 minutes. These figures also assume that the runner can not only run for 60 minutes but also remain within his or her aerobic training zone while doing so, continuing to burn fat. This is unrealistic for most people.

For every individual, there is a particular point at which we can no longer continue to work aerobically—that is, supply oxygen at the rate it is required. At this point, we then start to use the anaerobic energy system, which does not burn fat and in turn produces lactic acid in the muscle. This causes muscle soreness, which eventually stops the muscles from contracting. Whether or not you should walk or run to burn more fat, therefore, depends largely on your fitness level and on how long you are able to exercise.

When we compare walking and running over 20 minutes instead of 60, we can see that the difference between total calories burned and the percentage of fat calories burned is not so great:

	Walking	Running
Time	20 minutes	20 minutes
Total Calories	90	226
% Fat Calories	60	40
Total Fat Calories	54	90

A difference of 36 calories is negligible, especially when you consider that the calories you burn up after exercise are the most significant. Any exercise that you can sustain for 20 minutes or more will increase your metabolic rate for several hours afterward. If running is suitable for you, great; if not, no problem—just walk or do whatever you can.

In addition to this, you should remember that the total amount of calories burned will vary from one individual to another, according to the total body weight and the amount of lean body mass. One pound of muscle will require approximately 40 calories per day in order to function—excluding exercise. The more you exercise, the more calories the muscle will require—not just when you are exercising but throughout the day and night, as it repairs itself and starts to grow stronger. The result is a higher percentage of muscle on our bodies, so we burn more calories when we work out. This in turn means we burn more calories throughout the day and night, and so the cycle goes on. All these extra calories have to come from somewhere, and provided you are not eating more than you need, they will come from the body's fat stores—the perfect way to lose weight.

EVERYDAY EXERCISE

It is important not to get too bogged down with worrying about which exercise burns the most fat while you are working out. It is the total number of calories you burn in just staying alive that will influence how much or how little fat you burn. Only a small percentage of the calories you burn comes from exercise, compared with the amount burned just keeping you alive.

The exercise programs set out in this book include both aerobic and anaerobic exercises in order to stimulate the fat cells into releasing more fat (see Chapter 4), to replace muscle tissue and to increase the total amount of fat calories burned throughout the day—and night. What is vital, however, is that you adapt the program to suit you. For example, when choosing your aerobic activity, it is important to find something that you like to do and are able to do for at least 20 minutes—more if possible. You may find that power walking is a comfortable yet challenging workout for you if walking at a normal pace is not enough and running is too much. When power walking, you need to take much longer strides and use your arms and upper body to help you with the momentum. You should use as many of your muscles as possible and not just your legs.

Your body does not know the difference between providing energy for vacuuming and providing energy for an aerobics class. When the muscles start to work, the brain receives messages telling it to increase the supply of oxygen. This is the responsibility of the heart, which then has to pump faster to meet the increased demands. Here is a list of everyday activities that you probably do regularly, to show you that you really are burning up calories all day long:

Activity	Calories per Minute
driving a car	2.8
making beds	3.4
cleaning windows	3.7
sweeping floors	3.9
ironing	4.2
raking the lawn	4.7
weeding the garden	5.6
walking up stairs	10.0 or more

You can, therefore, make a considerable difference in the amount of calories you burn simply by being more active in everyday life.

CHAPTER 6

Perfecting Proportions

Designing Your Exercise Program

In order to maximize the amount of fat you burn from your body and to make sure that it stays off, you must include both aerobic and strength work in your exercise program.

As you start to exercise more regularly, you will see your shape changing and you will also have more energy. How quickly you start to see and feel these benefits will depend on several factors. For one, it will depend upon how hard you work. The improvements will occur in direct proportion to the level of overload (challenge) that you place on your body's systems. Complete beginners will achieve benefits from almost any level of exercise—even a gentle walk may be enough to cause the body to change. It will also depend on how often you exercise. You will need to commit yourself to regular times during the week; the more you do, the quicker you will improve—within reason. Finally it will depend on how long you spend exercising. If you want an aerobic workout, you should allow 30 minutes or more as you will need to warm up, stretch and cool down. The toning exercises, however, can be done in 15 minutes or less.

We can put these three factors into practice by using a FIT checklist:

Frequency = how often?
Intensity = how hard?
Time = how long?

At the end of each week, you must check your FIT list to make sure that you have achieved your goals. Fill in the chart as you design your own exercise regimen, so that you set aside time in advance to exercise. If you wait for a spare half an hour to come along, it never will—you have to *make* time!

	Aerobic	*Toning*	*Combination*
Frequency	Monday and Thursday	Wednesday and Friday	Saturday
Intensity	65%		65–75%
Time	30 minutes	15 minutes	60 minutes

By using the chart, you can schedule your exercise sessions and see in advance exactly what commitment you need to give to your program. It is vital that you write it down. If something is in your head, it is a dream, a wish or a hope; once it is written down, it becomes a commitment toward achieving your goal. Get your diary out *now* and schedule your workouts for this week. Make sure you do this at the start of every week.

THE AEROBIC WORKOUT

In order to work aerobically, your heart needs to be pumping blood and oxygen through your body at the same rate as they are being used. In simple terms, this means that you should be slightly breathless but not gasping. It is impossible to set a level of exercise that is going to be the same for everyone, so you will need to estimate how hard you are working. As mentioned previously, this can be done by taking your age and working out your maximum training heart rate by deducting your age from 220. An easier method is to use a **perceived rate of exertion (PRE) scale**, which gives you guidelines as to how you should be feeling. I have devised a simplified version of the PRE scale, which is much easier to follow:

Level 1	No effort
Level 2	Slight effort
Level 3	Effort required
Level 4	Rate of breathing starts to increase
Level 5	Slightly breathless; starting to perspire
Level 6	Breathless but comfortable; perspiring freely
Level 7	More breathless; still able to speak short sentences
Level 8	More breathless; able to speak only a few words
Level 9	Very breathless; unable to speak; feeling tired
Level 10	Very breathless; heavy legs; unable to continue

You should always begin with a warming-up period before you start the activity itself. This should include smaller movements using the same muscles that are going to be challenged when you are working out. For example, walking is a good warm-up exercise if you are going to power walk or jog. You should also include stretches for the leg muscles, as shown on pages 92–95. By the end of the warm-up, you should be feeling about level 4; you are now ready to begin your aerobic workout, and you should time it from this point. As you start to work a little harder, you should reach approximately level 6 or 7. This will ensure that you are well within your aerobic training zone and that you are burning fat. You should continue to exercise at this level for as long as is comfortable.

THE BENEFITS

The center of aerobic exercise is the heart, but it also involves many other important organs and systems. Any system of the body that is challenged will start to improve in efficiency. Aerobic exercise will, therefore, improve the efficiency of the heart, the respiratory system and the muscles used, as well as increase metabolism. When aerobic fitness improves, there is a real sense of well-being and an enhancement of mental health.

The heart is a muscle, and like any other muscle, it can grow stronger and, therefore, do more work with less effort. Imagine a weightlifter picking up a heavy weight and lifting it several times. Compare that with someone who doesn't exercise and who probably is unable to pick up a heavy weight at all. The weightlifter has stronger muscles, and we can train our hearts in the same way. The way in which we train aerobically differs from the way we strengthen other muscles in our bodies. We do not want to be able to occasionally do something really strenuous with our hearts for a short period of time; we want our hearts to get stronger so that they can beat more easily at a faster rate for a longer period. This form of training is called **endurance training**.

One of the ways in which the heart adapts to endurance training is that it increases slightly in size, which means it can pump more blood with every heartbeat—this is called **stroke volume**. Imagine two sponges: one small face sponge and one large bath sponge. If you had a leak or a puddle of water in a cupboard and used the two sponges to soak it up, you would, of course, see a marked difference between the efficiency of the two. The small sponge would fill up quickly, and when you squeezed it out, not much water would pass through it. You would be soaking and wringing it out very quickly to try to get rid of the water. On the other hand, if you used the big sponge, it would soak up more water, and when you squeezed it out, you would be able to pass a lot more water through it. The overall rate would be slower, however, because it would take more time to fill up and to empty. In other words, it would be pumping more slowly, *but* it would clean the water up more quickly and with less effort. It is logical to calculate that the small sponge will wear out very quickly due to overuse, while the life span of the big sponge will be much longer. As your heart increases in size and stroke volume, it will be doing more work with less effort. All your muscles will receive a healthy supply of oxygen and you will feel fitter.

Circulation is the process by which the blood is delivered to the muscles and into the cells, using a network of blood vessels. These blood vessels get gradually smaller and smaller until they become tiny capillaries. At this point, the oxygen literally hops off into the cells and carbon dioxide—a waste product of aerobic energy production—hops on and is carried, via the heart, back to the lungs, where it can be expelled when we breathe out. As we improve the efficiency of our hearts, we also improve the efficiency of our capillary networks. This means that there are more capillaries passing oxygen into the cells. With all this going on, it is hardly surprising that we start to feel more energetic.

There is no doubt that aerobic exercise is one of the best ways to strengthen your heart and to reduce the risk of heart disease and many other associated diseases. The good news is that anyone can do it. Aerobic exercise adds years to your life and life to your years.

CHOOSE YOUR EXERCISE

Because of the obvious limitations of exercising from a book, I am going to suggest that you choose your aerobic exercise from the following list. Choose two aerobic activities and do these twice per week. Make sure you use your exercise chart to schedule them so that you don't keep putting them off. Think of your exercise sessions as appointments that you *must* keep.

Power Walking
This involves both taking longer strides than you do when you walk normally and moving your arms as well as your legs, so that you can build up some momentum.

Jogging

Do this at a comfortable level that you can maintain. If you start to get breathless and unable to speak, reduce to a power walk. Make sure you wear some good running shoes, particularly if you are running on a concrete surface.

Swimming

When swimming, make sure that you use your legs as well as your arms. Try keeping your arms by your sides and just using your legs for some of the time. It doesn't really matter which stroke you use; choose the most comfortable for you, or better still, vary it every few lengths.

Cycling

Cycle at a comfortable level and try to choose a route that you can manage without stopping. Make sure you know what is around the corner. It may feel great going down a hill, but don't forget that you will have to get up the other side. Always wear a safety helmet and make sure that your bike is in good working order before you leave.

Stationary Cycling

This is one of the few workouts where it is possible to take your pulse rate fairly accurately. Pedal for at least five minutes, until you can feel you are perspiring and slightly breathless. Now take your pulse to see how hard you are working, using the maximum training heart rate guidelines. If you get bored, try putting the bike in front of the television and watching a video or a favorite program.

Stair Climbing

Step machines are relatively new, but very valuable, additions to home exercise equipment. As with stationary bikes, you can place them in front of the television or exercise while listening to music. They are available with frames to hold on to, or in smaller versions that have just the footpads. If possible, go for the larger variety, as the range of leg movements is greater. If not, make sure you try to use your arms as well.

Bench Stepping

Bench stepping involves stepping up and down on a small bench. Always choose a step that has adjustable heights since you may need to start out at four or six inches, as opposed to the maximum height of eight inches. Most steps come with an instructional video—if your step doesn't, you should buy one in order to ensure you are using a good technique. Although the step has been associated with knee injuries, improper step techniques have been responsible in almost all cases. Practiced properly, it is an excellent form of cardiovascular exercise. You could also join a step class, but make sure that the instructor teaches you properly.

Rowing

Rowing machines can be used for an excellent overall workout using lots of muscles. Recent studies have shown using a rowing machine to be one of the best forms of exercise for preventing osteoporosis (brittle bones) because it challenges muscles and puts stress on the bones, stimulating healthy bone-cell production.

Attending Aerobics Classes

Exercising in a group setting can often be more motivating than solo exercise. Do make sure, however, that the class you choose is at the appropriate level for you. Don't start off with the advanced class or one that is too heavily choreographed because you may not enjoy it. Make sure the aerobics section of the class lasts at least 20 minutes before going on to toning work. If toning work is included in the class, it will be a good combination workout.

You can vary your aerobic workout regularly. If you haven't exercised for a while, try different things until you find something that you enjoy. It doesn't matter what you do as long as you do something. Remember: Your heart doesn't know the difference between stepping and rowing; it just knows that it needs to work harder to pump more oxygen to the muscles. So the more muscles you are using, the better. Use the PRE scale to monitor how you are feeling. To stay within your aerobic threshold you should not go above level 7.

TONING EXERCISES (MUSCLE FITNESS)

Toning exercises are often referred to as strength work. Unfortunately this puts many people off since they associate strength with heavy weights and bulky muscles. This is not the case, however. It is possible to have a strength workout just using your body as resistance. This means altering your position in order to make the exercise harder or easier. As with all aspects of fitness, we tend to think of extremes, so visions of Olympic weightlifters spring to mind when we use the word "strength." Of course, these athletes do have to lift heavy weights and to train very hard to achieve their desired end result—but our desired result is quite different. We just want to strengthen our muscles so that they can support the weight of our skeletons and frames, to allow us to move and to accomplish everyday tasks more easily. The weightlifter ultimately has to lift a weight, so that is what he or she trains with. We, on the other hand, need to lift only our bodies or relatively light weights, so that's what we train with.

THE BENEFITS

As explained in Chapter 2, we lose muscle naturally as we get older. It literally wastes away, making us weaker. This is a natural process of aging that we cannot halt completely. We can, however, drastically reduce the rate at which it takes place, simply by using our muscles more. How sad it would be to reach retirement and not have the physical ability to enjoy the long-awaited fruits of years of hard work. Strength reaches a peak during our early 20s and then starts to decline. With exercise, however, it hardly declines at all. Muscular strength is just as important to overall health as aerobic fitness—only in a different way.

Complaints of back pain seem to have reached epidemic proportions. Numerous surveys have shown that an enormous number of people suffer from back pain at some point in their lives and that weak muscles are most commonly to blame. There is a balance between the front and the back of the body that must be maintained in order to ensure correct posture. Strong abdominal muscles are very important to ensuring stability of the spine. We should also work the muscles in the back, so that together the two muscle groups can hold us upright and allow the spine to move without suffering from stress.

Think of the spine as a pile of dominoes balanced one on top of the other. If you change the position of one near the bottom of the pile, it will affect the stability of the dominoes at the top. For the pile to remain stable, it is also important to balance them all correctly. Our spine is set in a delicate alignment and, unlike the dominoes, is S-shaped. This enables it to withstand maximum stress and impact. Any forces that strike at the feet are passed up the spine and need to be dissipated or reduced to prevent the vibrations from reaching the brain. This is why correct technique and appropriate footwear are so important when running. If you are heavy-footed as your foot strikes the ground, the shock it has to pass on is much greater, and therefore, the risk of injury much higher.

Osteoporosis, a disease in which bones become thin and brittle, is becoming more common as more people are living longer. Until recently it was thought of as a natural process of aging and believed to be both unavoidable and untreatable. Thankfully we now know much more about it, and more research is currently under way. What we have learned already is that there are ways to help prevent osteoporosis and that exercise is the key. When we contract a muscle, it pulls on a bone, causing movement. For example, if you bend your elbow, your biceps muscle literally pulls the bones in your lower arm closer to the bones in your upper arm. As it does this, it puts stress on the bone to which it is attached—rather like a tug-of-war team, where the anchor man withstands maximum stress from the pull of the rope. Because he doesn't want to move, he digs his heels in to provide a more stable base. The pull of a muscle on a bone means that the bone needs to withstand the stress of that pulling force, so it produces a higher rate of bone growth in order to prevent any weakening. Controlled strength exercises, such as those shown in this chapter, can put enough stress on the bone to stimulate improvements and reduce the risk of suffering from this terrible, debilitating disease.

Men and women have different potentials for building strength. Men are naturally more muscular due to a hormone called testosterone. The presence of this hormone also means that if they do strength work, they will increase the size of their muscles. Women, on the other hand, don't have the same potential to build muscle bulk. Many women are, however, put off by strength training because they fear developing big muscles. This fear is unfounded. Some female bodybuilders

87

have achieved big muscles only by taking testosterone supplements or similar substances and by using very heavy weights.
They also often develop other characteristics such as deep
voices. So if you are worried about building big muscles, don't
be—the exercises devised in this book are designed to
improve muscle tone and not increase muscle size, and there
is no testosterone included in the diet! The only muscle tissue
you will be building will be to replace the muscle tissue that
you have been losing for years.

So many things we do every day require strength. On a
typical day off, for example, I usually do the following: take
my three children to school; do some housework (moving
chairs and other furniture to vacuum behind them); carry
baskets of laundry upstairs and downstairs; and venture
around the supermarket. Shopping for a family of five, two
dogs and a cat is enough to fill any cart to the brim. I use
almost all of my muscles trying to steer the shopping cart
through the aisles without crashing into anyone, and then, of
course, the groceries need to be loaded into the car, unloaded
at the other end and put away. Next it's time to pick up the
children and walk the dogs, throwing sticks and balls across a
field for the dogs, before going home to cook dinner. When I
actually take time to analyze my activities throughout the day,
I see I am using my muscles all the time—so they need to be
strong.

On a typical working day, I am on the go all the time. At
the health and fitness club, I teach fitness classes and help
people around the gym all day, so the number of calories I can
burn in one day is very high for someone of my size. I have to
make sure that I eat well so that I have enough energy for my
muscles to do all this work, and I must also make sure that the
exercise program I do myself is well-balanced so that my
posture is good and I am less likely to suffer an injury.

As explained several times in this book, the main advantage of strength training for weight loss is that the increase in muscle tissue and tone (lean body mass, or LBM) means that we will burn more calories all day—not just when we are exercising. Take the list of things that I might do in a day off, for example. Because my ratio of LBM is good since I exercise regularly, I am burning more calories even when I do the shopping. My posture is good, and I have drastically reduced my risk of suffering from osteoporosis. By following the exercise programs in this book, you can achieve all these things for yourself.

HOW HARD YOU WORK

You want to strengthen your muscles to help you in everyday life, so you don't need to lift heavy weights and suffer resulting pain. With aerobic exercises, you should always feel comfortable and able to do more; with strength exercises, you should feel really challenged by the end of each set. When you do the exercises—although I have suggested the number of repetitions you should do—you may need to vary this to suit your own ability. If you are doing ten repetitions of something and then stopping, that represents one set. At the end of the set, if you feel as if you could have done a few more, then you have not worked hard enough. If you don't really challenge the muscle, it won't improve. If ten is the absolute maximum you can do and the last one is painful, then you are working too hard and should stop at eight or nine.

There is a difference between fatigue and failure. Fatigue means that the muscle feels tired after you have completed the set and that you feel you have really achieved something. This is the level you want to aim for. Failure means that the last exercise (repetition) in the set was painful and that you couldn't complete it properly. You should avoid this stage since your muscles are likely to be very sore a day or two later and you may injure yourself. It is very important when doing strength work that you work to fatigue, not failure.

The toning exercises I have devised can easily be done at home. They should take approximately 15 minutes or less, including some warm-up and stretching exercises. There are two programs, although some of the exercises are the same in both. The programs have been carefully designed to balance muscle strength evenly to promote good posture.

THE COMBINATION WORKOUT

I have included a combination workout that you should do at least once per week. A combination workout is a program including both aerobic and muscular strength work to promote overall fitness. Simply choose one of the aerobic exercises suggested and one of the toning workouts. For example, you could start with a warm-up followed by 20 minutes or more of power walking, and then come home to do the toning exercises, followed by a good stretch. I suggest you allow an hour for this, although you may find you can do it in less.

The exercise program I have given you—aerobics twice per week, strength twice per week and one combination workout—is enough for you to really see and feel the benefits. If you practice this program conscientiously and follow the diet, you will succeed. If you choose to exercise more frequently, that is fine, but make sure you have one or two days per week when you do no exercise, in order to allow the body to rest and recover. Exercise is clearly a good thing. If you go over sensible limits, however, it can be a bad thing, and you may end up feeling run-down and unwell. I hope you have learned from reading this book that losing weight should not mean going through torture sessions and that you can achieve really good results without breaking the pain barrier.

Once you have achieved your goal, you will need to exercise regularly to maintain it, although you can reduce the frequency to two or three times per week. I recommend one toning workout, one aerobic and one combination.

WARMING UP

Before commencing any kind of workout, you should always begin with a warm-up. This is essential because it reduces the risk of injury, which can be quite high if the body is not prepared properly. The type of warm-up exercise you should do depends on the kind of exercises you will be doing in your workout.

THE AEROBIC WARM-UP

The purpose of the aerobic warm-up is to raise the pulse to a comfortable level so that you can exercise safely within your training zone. For example, if you are power walking, you should begin by walking at a normal pace and circle your shoulders slowly until you feel your heart rate has increased and you have reached level 4 on the PRE scale. (See pages 79–80.) The principle is the same for all the aerobic activities— that is, start swimming, cycling, stepping or rowing at a gentle pace and then gradually increase it. When you feel your pulse rate has achieved level 4 (PRE scale), you should then do the following stretches:

Front of Thigh (Quads)

Using a wall for balance, place one foot in your hand and ease the leg back slowly until the knee is behind the hip. Keep the hips square, pull your abdomen in to support your back and tilt your pelvis under. You should feel the stretch across the front of the hip and down the front of the thigh. Hold for 8 to 10 seconds, then repeat with the other leg.

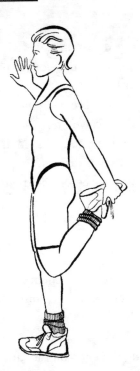

Back of Thigh (Hamstrings)

Stand with one foot in front of the other, as if you had taken a generous stride forward, and transfer all of your weight to your back leg; bending the leg, sit down into the stretch. Support your body weight with both hands on the thigh of the bent leg and tilt the pelvis so that the base of your spine is inclined toward the ceiling. Keep the hips square. You should feel this down the back of the straight leg, from the hip to just below the knee. Hold for 8 to 10 seconds, then repeat with the other leg.

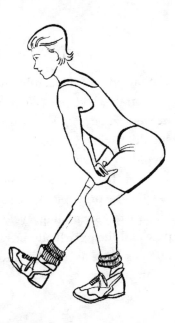

Calf (Gastrocnemius)

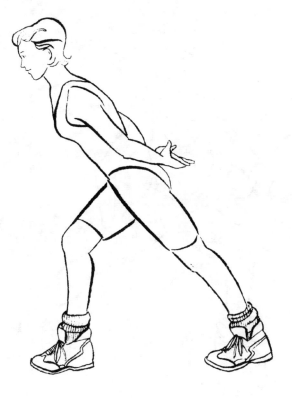

Stand with one foot in front of the other, as if you had taken a generous stride forward. Bend the front leg and transfer the body weight forward; make sure that the heel of the back foot is on the floor and that the toes are facing forward. Press the hips forward to ensure that your body forms a diagonal line from your head to your toes. Hold for 8 to 10 seconds, then repeat with the other leg.

Inner Thigh (Adductors)

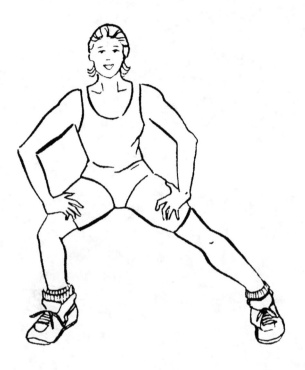

Stand with your feet wide apart. Bend one leg and transfer the body weight over to this leg. Make sure that your knee does not go over the line of your toe. You should be able to see your foot—if not, your feet are too close together. Keep the hips square to the front. You should feel this on the inside thigh of the straight leg. Hold for 8 to 10 seconds, then repeat with the other leg.

Outer Thigh (Abductors)

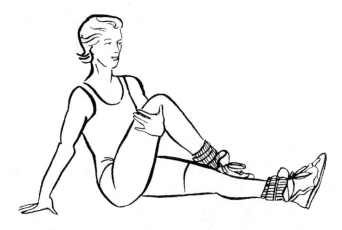

Sit on the floor with the left leg straight in front of you. Bend the right knee and cross it over the left leg. Keep the right hand on the floor, and using the left hand, pull the right knee gently toward you. You should feel the stretch in the outside of the right thigh. Hold for 8 to 10 seconds, then repeat with the other leg.

Back (Erector Spinae)

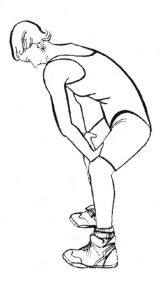

Stand with your feet slightly wider than hip width apart; bend the knees and lower into a squatting position. Place your hands just above your knees and support your body weight in your arms. Pull the abdomen in and tuck your head and pelvis under to arch the spine. You should feel this all the way down the back. Hold for 8 to 10 seconds, then repeat.

THE TONING WARM-UP

It is not necessary to raise the pulse for toning work, but you should mobilize the joints that you are going to use. Repeat the following exercises 8 to 10 times:

Shoulder Circles

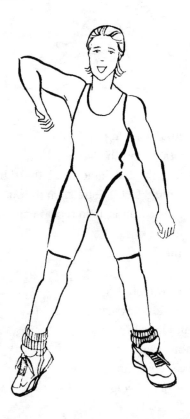

Stand with the feet apart and transfer your weight from side to side. As you do this, circle alternate shoulders. Start with small circles and increase the size of the circles gradually until you are doing full-arm circles.

Side Bends

Stand with your feet hip width
apart. Keeping the hips square
to the front, lean slowly down
to each side as far as is comfortable.

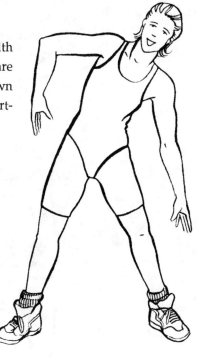

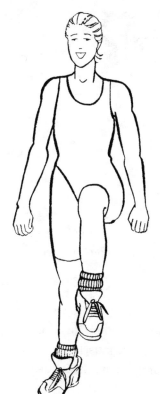

Knee Lifts

Raise alternate knees to hip height,
pulling the abdomen in as you lift to
support the back.

Hamstring Curls

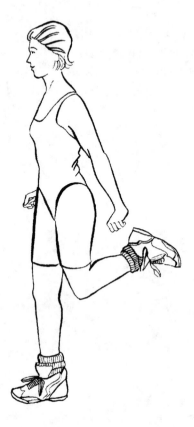

With feet apart, transfer the body weight from one leg to the other. Kick back with alternate legs so that your heel comes toward your bottom.

After you have done the mobility exercises above, you will need to do the stretches shown for the aerobic warm-up. In addition to these, you should also stretch some other muscles that you will be using during the toning section by doing the following exercises:

Chest (Pectorals)

Stand with your feet apart and place your hands on your bottom. Gently squeeze your elbows together behind your back. You should feel the stretch across the front of the chest and the shoulders. Hold for 8 to 10 seconds.

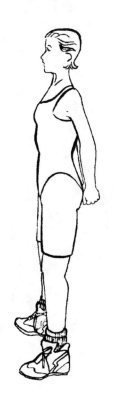

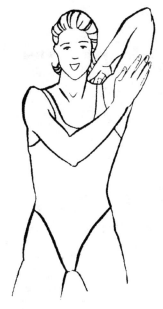

Upper Arm (Triceps)

Reach up with one arm, bend the elbow and touch the back of your shoulder with your hand. Using the other arm, gently push the arm back. You should feel the stretch down the back of the arm. Hold for 8 to 10 seconds.

Upper Back (Trapezius and Rhomboids)

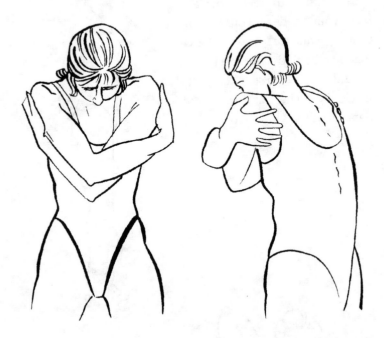

Stand with your feet apart. Fold your arms in front of you and hug your body, reaching around your shoulders with your hands. You should feel the stretch across the upper back and the back of the shoulders. Hold for 8 to 10 seconds.

COOLING DOWN

After any form of exercise, it is important to cool down. As with warming up, this helps prevent injury and muscle soreness.

THE AEROBIC COOLDOWN

When you are working aerobically, the heart is pumping blood through the body much faster than it does normally in order to supply more oxygen to the muscles. If you suddenly stop exercising—going from running to standing still, for example—the heart continues pumping blood to the muscles at this elevated rate. The muscles, however, are not contracting and thus are not pushing the blood back to the heart and the brain, so you may feel giddy or even pass out. You should reduce the intensity of the movements gradually, until you can feel your heart rate slowing down. For example, if you are running, slow down to a gentle jog, then to a brisk walk and, finally, to a slow walk before stopping. The amount of time it takes to cool down depends on your fitness level. Initially it may take four to five minutes, but as your body becomes used to exercise, you will be able to reduce your pulse rate in two to three minutes.

Another reason for cooling down is to give the muscles the chance to flush out any lactic acid. The cooldown brings new blood into the muscle, forcing the used blood out. The waste products—which include lactic acid—are then carried back to the liver where they are broken down and disposed of. If you have ever experienced muscle soreness after a workout, it is more likely to be because you did not cool down properly than because you were working too hard—although working too hard can also cause pain and soreness a day or two after exercise.

COOL-DOWN STRETCHES

After any kind of workout, you should stretch the muscles you have been using to prevent muscle stiffness and promote flexibility. Repeat the stretches you did before the workout.

TONING PROGRAM 1

Front of Thigh (Quads)

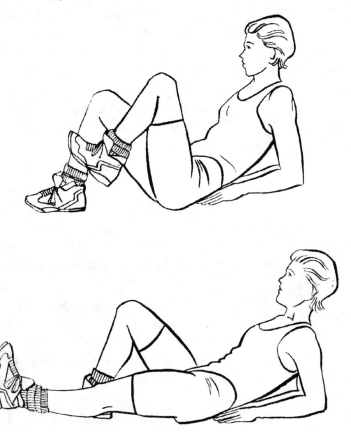

From a sitting position, lean back so that you are supporting your weight on your elbows. Keep your abdomen pulled in tightly to support your back and bend one knee so that your foot is close to your bottom. Bend the other leg in toward your

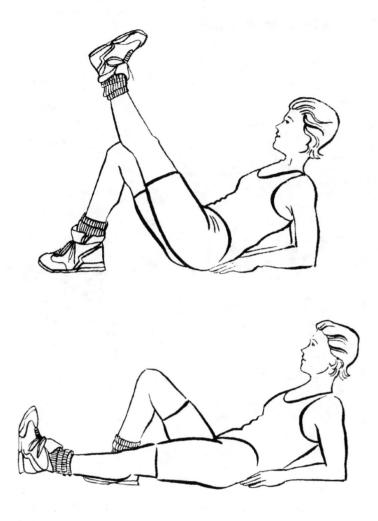

chest; extend it, keeping it just off the floor, then lift and lower it carefully. Repeat the whole movement.

Suggested repetitions: 10 to 12 each leg

Back of Thigh (Hamstrings)

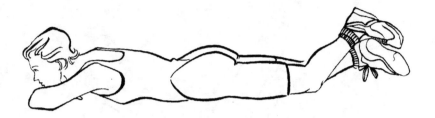

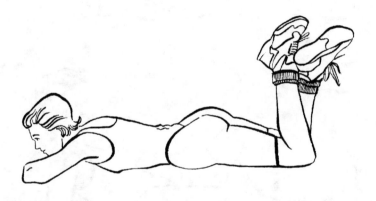

Lie facedown on the floor, cross your ankles and resist with the top leg as you bend the lower leg. You can add as much or as little pressure as is comfortable.

Suggested repetitions: 8 to 10 each leg

Outer Thigh (Abductors)

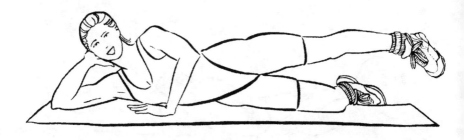

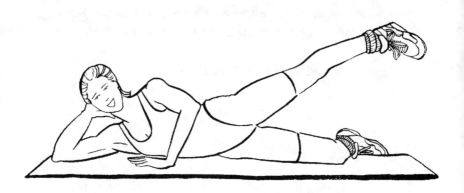

Lie on your side, supporting your neck in your hand. Bend the lower leg and straighten the top leg. Make sure that your hips are square to the front, then raise and lower the top leg, leading with the heel. Aim to touch the toe on the floor each time you lower your leg.

Suggested repetitions: 10 to 12 each leg

Bottom (Glutei)

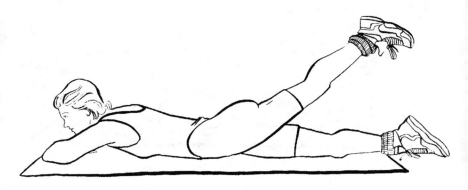

Lie facedown on the floor, resting your head in your hands. Keep the hips square and lift alternate legs. Make sure you do not roll your hips.

Suggested repetitions: 14 to 16 each leg

Abdomen (Rectus Abdominus)

Lie on your back with your knees bent. Press your abdomen down into the floor, and as you do so, curl your ribs toward your hips. Lower yourself back down and repeat. Think of it as a curling movement and not a lift. You can select a hand position that is most comfortable for you, either across the chest or beside the head to make it more difficult. You may need to support your neck by placing your hand on the back of your neck and allowing your head to rest on your forearm as you curl up.

Suggested repetitions: 10 to 12

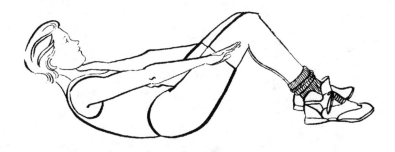

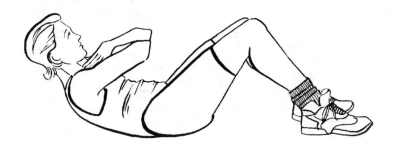

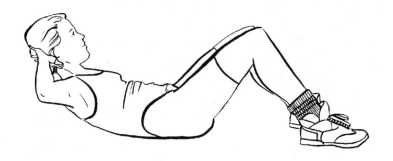

Upper Back (Trapezius and Rhomboids)

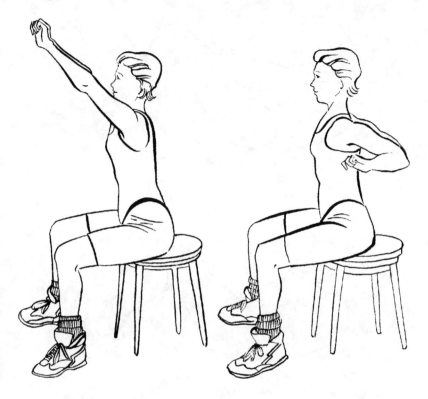

Sit upright on a chair, close to the front. Reach upward and forward. Pull your arms back and down in a diagonal line, trying to squeeze your shoulder blades together as you do so. Reach up and repeat. You can hold light weights such as cans of food to make this more difficult as you grow stronger.

Suggested repetitions: 10 to 12

Upper Arm (Biceps)

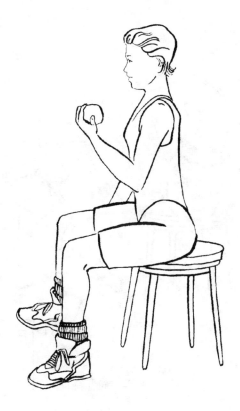

While sitting upright on a chair, hold a light weight in each hand (a can of food, for example). Raise your arms slightly in front of you and bend each arm alternately. Keep your elbows close to your body.

Suggested repetitions: 16 to 18 each arm

Back of Arm (Triceps)

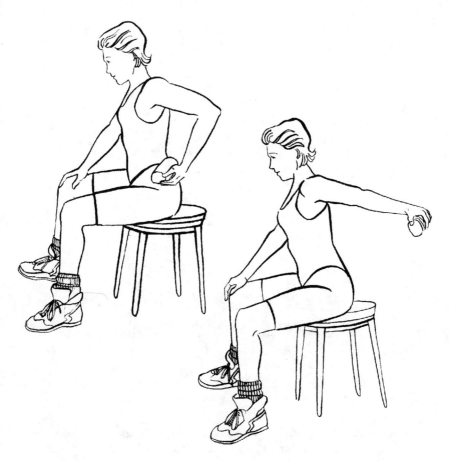

While sitting slightly forward on a chair, place your hands by your sides behind you. Bend both arms so that your hands are hip height and your elbows are well behind you. Keeping the top of your arm still, straighten one elbow, then bend it back to the original position and repeat with the other arm. Keep your abdomen pulled in to support your back. Again, cans of food may be used to make this more difficult.

Suggested repetitions: 12 to 14 each arm

TONING PROGRAM 2

Leg (Quads, Glutei and Hamstrings)

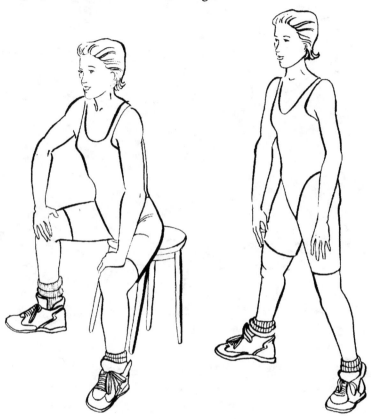

Sit on a chair with your feet slightly apart. Place your hands on your thighs and stand up. As you do so, press your hips forward. From the standing position, bend the knees and slowly lower yourself back down into a sitting position. As you get stronger, you can do this without the chair, but make sure that your bottom doesn't go below your knees as you squat down.

Suggested repetitions: 10 to 12

Inner Thigh (Adductors)

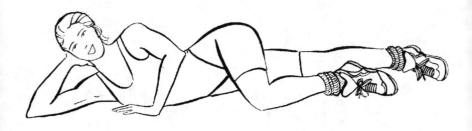

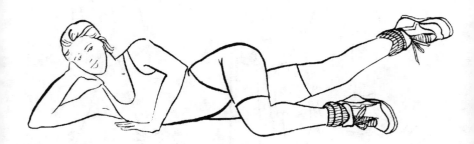

Lie on your side with your top leg bent across so that your knee is level with your hips. Straighten the lower leg so that your heel is in line with your hips, not in front or behind. Keeping this leg straight, lift it as high as possible without turning the hips, and then lower it without putting the weight back onto the floor. After you have finished the whole set, repeat using the other leg.

Suggested repetitions: 8 to 10

Abdomen (Rectus Abdominus)

Follow the instructions on pages 106–107.

112

Chest (Pectorals)

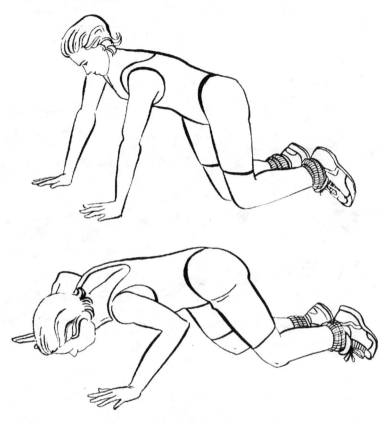

On your hands and knees, place your hands slightly wider than your shoulders, making sure that your chin is in line with your fingers. Pull your abdomen in to support your back and bend your arms slowly, lowering your nose almost to the floor. Straighten your arms and push back up again.

If this is too difficult for you or is painful for your wrists, lie on your back on the floor with your arms bent (hold cans of food to make it more challenging) and bring your forearms together. Lower and repeat.

Suggested repetitions: 6 to 8

Back (Erector Spinae)

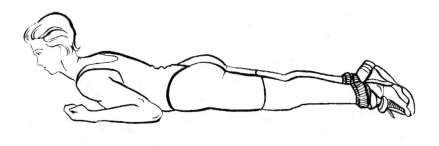

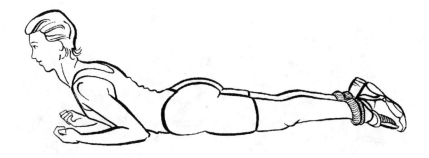

Lie on your front with your arms bent close to your body, placing your hands slightly wider than your shoulders with palms
turned up. Using the muscles in your back, raise your shoulders
slightly off the floor. Your elbows will provide stability but
should not do the work. Lower slowly and repeat.

Suggested repetitions: 6 to 8

Waist (Obliques)

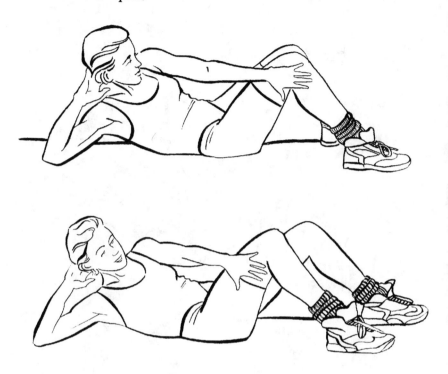

Lie on your back with your knees bent and your feet slightly apart. Keeping the hips still, lift and turn your upper body so that you touch the outside of the opposite thigh with your hand. You may need to support the neck with the other hand as you do this. You must aim to curl the ribs toward the hips and turn at the same time, without rolling the hips. Lower slowly and carefully and repeat.

Suggested repetitions: 8 each side

Shoulder (Anterior Deltoid)

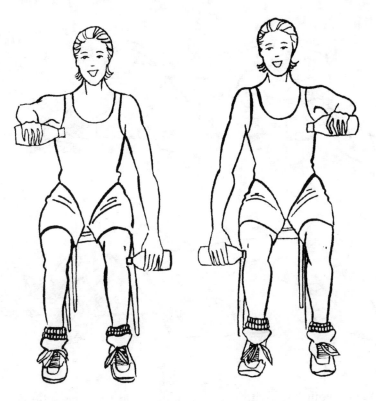

While sitting on a chair and holding a light weight in each hand (a can of food, for example), pull your abdomen in to support your back. Raise alternate arms in front of you to just above shoulder height. Lower slowly.

Suggested repetitions: 12 to 14 each arm

Shoulder (Superior Deltoid)

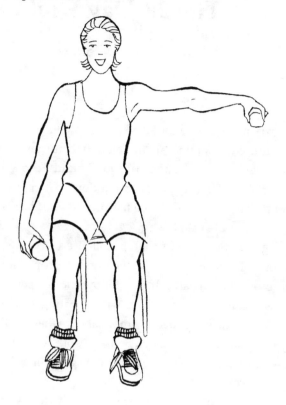

While sitting on a chair as before, raise alternate arms to the side. Keep your hands in line with your body, not in front or behind. Lift each arm to just above shoulder height and lower slowly.

Suggested repetitions: 12 to 14 each arm

CHAPTER 7

The 28-Day Diet

The Recipes for Success

As explained throughout the book, it is vital to ensure that the food you eat contains all the essential nutrients your body requires in order to function properly and keep you in good health. When dieting, people often don't eat enough. Keep in mind that this practice can be harmful to your health and may actually promote weight gain.

A good diet is one that is balanced—that is, one that contains all the nutrients in the correct proportions to help ensure optimum health. If you follow the recipes in the plan, then you can rest assured you will be eating a balanced diet. However, now that you know more about what foods you need and in what quantities, you will be able to plan your own balanced diet, provided you stick to the guidelines I have established for you.

This 28-day diet plan has been carefully designed to ensure maximum nutritional content and maximum taste. So often we associate diets with tasteless and boring meals such as lettuce leaf sandwiches. In this book, however, you will find the recipes mouthwatering and delicious. My thanks to Sharman Thomson, a *cordon bleu* chef, for her expertise in helping me to select the right ingredients and cooking methods to ensure that every meal is delicious.

If you follow this plan, you will not only lose weight but also be more likely to stay in good health and feel full of vitality.

The plan is easy to follow and can be adapted to suit different tastes as well as different circumstances. There are, however, a few guidelines that you should follow strictly. These are all outlined below.

BREAKFAST—KICK-START THE METABOLISM

Always have breakfast—it is vital to get your metabolism going. Choose something from the following section.

CEREAL

Most people start the day with cereal, which can be very nutritious. You should, however, avoid the sugar-coated varieties, even if they are promoted as being low in fat. (Some low-fat cereals are actually coated with more sugar than the regular varieties.) Always check the label for this before you buy. Beware of refined cereals as well, as these have all undergone rigorous processing. Although many cereals advertise "fortified with vitamins and minerals," what this really means is that the cereals have been stripped of all their natural nutritional content in processing, and a few known nutrients have been replaced.

If you are used to sugar-coated cereals and don't like the taste of the bran cereals, try slowly weaning yourself off of the sweet ones. I was a frosted flakes fan for many years and gradually started to mix in some bran flakes. I started off with a mix of 80 percent frosted flakes and 20 percent bran flakes and worked my way down to bran flakes with some fruit to replace the sweet taste. Now that I have reeducated my palate, I usually have a hot cereal with bran and some chopped fruit, which sets me up for the day. If you prefer, you can also mix your cereal with low-fat yogurt or low-fat ricotta cheese instead of milk. This can really enhance the taste of the blander varieties.

Here are my recommendations for cereals:
- hot, whole-grain cereal (preferably organic, or grown without pesticides) with water and/or skim milk
- bran cereal with skim milk and a piece of fresh fruit, chopped
- two shredded wheat biscuits with skim milk, sweetened with honey (preferably organically produced) if necessary
- muesli with skim milk. Beware of brands that contain a large quantity of nuts, as these can be very high in fat. Always check the label before you buy.

If you don't like cereal:
- fresh fruit—two pieces of the fruit of your choice, peeled and cut into small pieces, with low-fat yogurt, ricotta cheese or skim milk. Alternatively, if you are eating breakfast on the run, take two pieces of fruit and a carton of juice (pure with no added sugar) with you to eat on the journey.
- toast—two slices of thickly cut whole-wheat bread. Do not spread with butter; have jam or honey instead (organic honey, if possible). Some people feel very bloated and suffer from constipation when they eat bread. This is quite common and can be due to an intolerance of wheat. If this applies to you, you may be able to tolerate white bread only; if you cannot, avoid bread altogether.

LIGHT LUNCHES

Always have lunch. If you don't have time to prepare some of the lunches I have included, then select some of the easier alternatives—for example, a sandwich—instead. This is also more practical if you take a packed lunch to work.

As you will see, I have included several soups on the lunch

menus. These recipes will make enough for several days for one person and can be frozen. You can make the soups thicker or thinner, according to preference, simply by using more or less stock. All soups should be served with a large whole-grain roll or a thick slice of whole-grain bread.

Where a sandwich or baked potato is shown, select one of the fillings listed below (use two or three slices of whole-grain bread for the sandwich):

- tuna fish (in spring water) with a pinch of fresh basil
- cottage cheese and pineapple
- salmon and cucumber
- salad with a touch (1/4 tsp) of horseradish
- cottage cheese with finely chopped celery and apple
- sardines (in tomato juice, not oil) and watercress
- snow peas and tomatoes finely chopped with 1/4 tsp of mixed-grain mustard
- hummus, cucumber and a pinch of dill
- watercress, grated carrots and cottage cheese
- cottage cheese, a finely chopped peach and 1/4 tsp mustard
- tuna fish (in spring water) with a pinch of coriander
- hummus with tomato and black pepper
- mixed bean salad, drained—as a baked potato topping only
- baked beans—as a baked potato topping only

HUMMUS

I have listed hummus above as a sandwich filling. However, many store-bought varieties are very high in fat (some contain as much as 85 percent fat), so I recommend that you make your own. It's very quick and easy to do—it takes about five minutes and can be kept in the refrigerator for about four days, or according to the date shown on the yogurt. You can adjust the texture a little by adding more or less yogurt. You will need:

13 oz chickpeas, blended (with a fork or in a blender or food
    processor) for a smoother texture
5 to 7 oz low-fat ricotta cheese or plain yogurt
pinch of black pepper and lemon juice, to taste
1 clove garlic, chopped

Mix all the ingredients together in a bowl and place in the refrigerator to cool.

YOUR EVENING MEAL

Try not to eat your evening meal too late. I have put the largest meal in the evening simply because that is the most common time for people to eat it. However, if it suits your timetable to eat your main meal at lunch, that's fine—in fact, it's preferable.

The recipes for the main meal serve four people. Obviously they can be halved for two people or you can freeze some of the meals (this is indicated at the top of the relevant recipes). As a working mother, I find it very useful to have some nutritious meals ready in the freezer as this stops the temptation to get takeout after a busy day when I feel too tired to cook.

As with the lunchtime menus, it's not essential that you have everything in the order shown. For example, if you dislike the recipe for a particular day, simply swap that meal for one you prefer from another day. I have included several fish recipes because fish is an excellent source of essential fatty acids. Even if you don't usually eat fish, try these recipes—they are delicious. You should eat fish at least once a week.

As you will see, the main meal does not state what you should serve with it as this is up to you. However, you must have either a large portion of salad or at least two vegetables

(lightly cooked) with every meal. You should also choose potatoes, rice (preferably brown) or pasta. It is very important that
you feel satisfied after each meal—if you do not, have low-fat
yogurt or low-fat ricotta cheese with some chopped fruit in it.

SALAD

I tend to make a large salad every four days and keep it in
an airtight container in the refrigerator. It will remain fresh,
provided the container you put it in is clean and dry. This saves
you from making up a salad every day, which can be time-
consuming. You can vary the ingredients in terms of quantities
and according to taste and what is available, but it must include
at least some, if not all, of the following:
- lettuce
- raw spinach leaves
- chopped broccoli
- chopped cauliflower
- snow peas
- bean sprouts (fresh)
- chopped or grated carrot
- chopped raw pepper
- sliced zucchini
- 1 1/2 tsp sesame seeds per salad bowl

FOR VEGETARIANS

I have included a vegetarian option for every meal containing
meat. I recommend that you eat the fish dishes; these are essential
to ensure an adequate intake of nutrients. If you do not eat fish,
simply select one of the other vegetarian options. I would urge
you, however, to seek professional nutritional advice, as you may
need to supplement some nutrients, particularly vitamin B_{12}.

THE DESSERT CART

As you will see, I have not included a dessert with meals as it is not essential. You should try to educate your palate not to expect something sweet after every meal. However, if you do want to have something simple after your meal, choose a low-fat yogurt, ricotta cheese or some fresh fruit. Alternatively, if you're planning a special meal, there are a few options listed below. Please remember, however, that just because these desserts are low in fat, it doesn't mean that you can eat twice as much. Give yourself a modest portion and don't have seconds.

Fat-Free Mousse • SERVES 2

A delicious and light dessert that will accompany any main meal beautifully. It can be made in any flavor—my personal favorites are pineapple and black cherry.

4 oz flavored instant gelatin
7 oz fat-free yogurt of the same flavor

1. Make the gelatin according to the instructions on the label and place in the refrigerator to cool.
2. When the gelatin is semi-set, whisk in the yogurt. Return to the refrigerator to cool fully before serving.

Rice Pudding • SERVES 2 TO 4

1 packet rice pudding
jam or honey (organic, if possible) or fresh fruit of your choice

1. Make the rice pudding according to the instructions on the packet using skim milk.
2. Sweeten with the jam or honey or stir in some chopped fruit as you serve.

Hot Fruit Salad • SERVES 4

2 medium bananas
10 oz canned mandarin oranges in fruit juice
2 large oranges, cut into segments
cinnamon, to taste
10 oz low-fat ricotta cheese

1. Place the fruit in a large frying pan or wok, add the juice from the mandarins and heat slowly.
2. Add the cinnamon and bring to a boil. Continue to boil until the juice has evaporated.
3. Serve immediately with the ricotta cheese.

Summer Fruit Flan • SERVES 4

3 eggs
3 oz sugar
3 oz flour
5 oz ricotta cheese
1 pint strawberries and/or raspberries

1. Preheat the oven to 300°F.
2. Break the eggs into a bowl and add the sugar.
3. Place the bowl inside a larger bowl containing freshly boiled water and whisk the eggs until very stiff. Remove the bowl from the water and continue to whisk until the bowl has completely cooled.
4. Sift the flour and fold into the eggs very carefully, a third at a time. Place the mixture in a 6-inch nonstick cake pan and bake in the oven for 10 to 15 minutes.
5. When the flan has cooled, slice off the top carefully so that the surface is level. Spread the ricotta cheese onto the surface and decorate with the fruit.

Upside-Down Cheesecake • SERVES 6

10 oz canned mandarin oranges or pineapple in juice
 (preferably not syrup)
1 packet gelatin
12 oz low-fat ricotta cheese
2 egg whites
8 low-fat graham crackers, crushed

1. Drain the fruit and pour the juice into a small bowl or cup.
   Fill a larger bowl with freshly boiled water and place the cup
   inside the bowl.
2. Allow the gelatin to dissolve in the juice. Remove the cup
   from the hot water and allow to cool.
3. Fold the drained fruit into the ricotta cheese and slowly pour
   in the gelatin/juice mixture.
4. Whisk the egg whites until they are very stiff and then fold
   them carefully into the mixture. Place this in an 8-inch
   loose-bottomed, nonstick pan and spread the crumbs over
   the top of the cheesecake. (It is not essential to use the
   crumbs. The cheesecake will be delicious as it is and, of
   course, lower in fat.)
5. Place in the refrigerator to cool and set before serving.

SUNDAY ROAST

I have not included a roast dinner in the plan, although the Sunday meals are substantial. (If you start the plan on a Monday, they will fall automatically on days 7, 14, 21 and 28.) If you would prefer to have a traditional Sunday roast, however, it is not a problem, provided you make a few alterations to the traditional way of cooking it. These are all outlined in the tips below.

The danger with a roast dinner is that we tend to pile our plates high and eat far more than we actually need. Be sensible when you serve yourself; don't take any more than you actually need to satisfy your hunger. Stuffing is not recommended, and if you feel you need a dessert, the fat-free mousse shown on page 124 makes an ideal light accompaniment your roast dinner.

My tips for cooking a healthy roast are:
- Select chicken or turkey and remove the skin before cooking. Place 1 level tsp tarragon and a generous pinch of mixed herbs inside the bird and lay it in a large roasting pan with a lid or foil to cover. Mix a cup of vegetable or chicken stock with hot water and pour into the roasting pan. Place a sheet of waxed paper over the bird and put the lid or foil back on to seal. Cook for the recommended time, then let stand for 5 to 10 minutes, keeping the lid on. Remove the meat, drain and carve.
- Peel and parboil the potatoes. Using a pastry brush, paint the bottom of a roasting pan very lightly with extra-virgin olive oil and put in the oven to heat. Sprinkle 1/2 to 1 tsp dried rosemary over the parboiled potatoes and place in the hot pan. Cook for up to an hour, turning at least once. Or sprinkle the potatoes with rosemary and then dry-roast them.

- Boil your vegetables—fresh vegetables of your choice and at least one dark green variety—in your usual way and save the water from the cooking for the gravy.
- To make your gravy, take a little of the stock from the chicken or turkey and place in a fat-separating pitcher. Let stand for 5 minutes in a cool place. Using the vegetable water, season to taste with a vegetable or chicken stock cube, add 2 tbsp of the meat stock (once it has separated from the fat) and stir over a low heat. Mix 1 to 2 tbsp cornstarch with some water and stir until it makes a smooth paste. Remove the gravy from the heat and add in the cornstarch slowly. Replace over low heat and continue to stir until the gravy reaches the desired consistency.

FRUIT

When planning your food for the day, you must include three pieces of fruit. This is very important as it ensures that you get adequate amounts of fiber and other nutrients. You can have the fruit either as part of a meal—chopped banana in your cereal, for example—or on its own as a snack between meals.

WHAT TO DRINK

Water is undoubtedly the best drink, particularly if you have a water filter. There is a lot of controversy over what and how much you should drink with a meal. Tea and coffee should definitely be avoided within 30 minutes either side of a meal, as they drastically reduce the amount of nourishment you can absorb from your food. Fruit juice is fine, provided it doesn't have added sugar—always check the label for details as clever marketing can be misleading. Even pure fruit juice is best diluted.

Drinks to avoid are those in cans, which are packed full of preservatives, sugar or artificial sweeteners. Don't be fooled just because the label says "sugar free." These drinks have absolutely no nutritional value whatsoever and can damage your teeth, not to mention your insides. Other drinks to watch out for are some fruit-flavored sodas, which are also packed with sugar and preservatives.

So-called energy drinks can be made easily and cheaply at home, without any of the additives: Dilute some fresh juice of your choice with water—about 30 percent juice, 70 percent water—add a pinch of salt and stir well. The only thing contained in these sport drinks that is of value is the salt (electrolytes), which helps to ensure that the body absorbs the fluid quickly. Most of all the body needs water—and not glucose or sugar—in order to keep on performing.

Throughout the day you should sip water regularly, every time you go into the kitchen at home or into the break room at work. Have a small glass of water even if you are not thirsty. If you are feeling thirsty, then your body is probably already 30 percent dehydrated.

ALCOHOL

The body cannot use alcohol for muscular work. In other words, it cannot be burned off and it also has little or no nutritional value. It makes sense, therefore, not to have too much of it. In this plan, I recommend a maximum of one glass of wine or spirits three or four times per week. This does not mean, however, that you can save up your allowance and have it all in one go on a Saturday night! If you do this, your total calories for that day will be excessive, and excess calories, no matter what foods they come from, end up as fat.

RECIPES

DAY 1

LUNCH

Pizza Bread • SERVES 1

7 oz canned tomatoes
1/2 small onion, chopped
1 tsp tomato puree
pinch of oregano (optional)
2 medium slices bread
1 oz cottage cheese

1. Simmer the tomatoes, onion, puree and oregano for approximately 10 minutes, until they are reduced to a thick puree.
2. Toast the bread on one side. Spread the mixture over the other side, then dot this lightly with the cottage cheese.
3. Broil for 1 to 2 minutes on low to moderate heat.

DINNER

Sweet-and-Sour Pork or Chicken • SERVES 4

2 cloves garlic, crushed
1/4 tsp chili powder
1 oz fresh gingerroot, peeled and chopped
12 oz chicken or pork, cut into cubes

1/2 tsp sesame oil
1 green pepper, diced
1 red pepper, diced
1 large onion, chopped
2 medium carrots, thinly sliced
3 slices fresh or canned pineapple, cubed

Sauce
4 tbsp white wine vinegar
2 tbsp cornstarch
2 tbsp soy sauce
1 oz brown sugar
2 tbsp tomato puree

1. Mix the garlic, chili and ginger with the meat, cover and place in the refrigerator for at least 2 hours.
2. Heat the sesame oil in a pan, add the meat and cook for several minutes, stirring continuously. Remove the meat and place in a dish.
3. Add the vegetables and the pineapple to the pan and stir-fry for 2 minutes. Remove and add to the meat.
4. To make the sauce, add 1 to 2 tbsp white wine vinegar to the cornstarch in a bowl to make a paste. Put the soy sauce, remaining vinegar, sugar and tomato puree into the pan and heat to just boiling. Pour this onto the cornstarch mixture and stir until all paste is dissolved.
5. Pour the sauce back into the pan, stirring constantly to make sure it's smooth. Return the meat and vegetables to the pan and cook with the sauce for 3 to 4 minutes. Serve immediately.

Vegetarian Option

Sweet-and-Sour Vegetables • SERVES 4

1/2 tsp sesame oil

4 oz mushrooms, sliced

1 medium zucchini, sliced

1 large carrot, chopped

1 large red pepper, chopped

6 oz broccoli florets

4 oz bean sprouts

2 cloves garlic, crushed

1/4 tsp chili powder

1 oz fresh gingerroot, peeled and chopped

Sauce

4 tbsp white wine vinegar

2 tbsp cornstarch

2 tbsp soy sauce

1 oz brown sugar

2 tbsp tomato puree

1. Heat the sesame oil, add the vegetables, garlic, chili powder and ginger and cook for several minutes, stirring continually. (Other vegetables may also be used, such as baby sweet corn and snow peas.) Remove the vegetables to a separate dish.
2. Make the sauce as described on the previous page.
3. Put the vegetables back into the pan with the sauce and cook for 3 to 4 minutes. Serve immediately.

DAY 2

LUNCH

Vegetable Soup • SERVES 4 • CAN BE FROZEN

2 medium potatoes, finely chopped
2 medium carrots, finely chopped
1 onion, finely chopped
1 leek, finely chopped
1 parsnip, finely chopped
1 to 2 cups water or vegetable stock
1 bay leaf
parsley, to taste
pinch of salt and pepper

1. Cover the vegetables with the water or stock. Add the bay leaf, parsley, salt and pepper.
2. Cook slowly (simmer) for 45 minutes. Blend in a blender or food processor until smooth and serve.

DINNER

Smoked Mackerel With Pasta • SERVES 4

4 large peppered, smoked mackerel fillets
2 tbsp lemon juice
1 tbsp capers, chopped
1 large sprig of basil, shredded
4 tbsp parsley, chopped
2 tbsp freshly snipped chives
1 lb pasta
5 oz low-fat ricotta cheese

1. Remove the skin and bones from the mackerel and flake the remaining meat. Mix in the lemon juice, capers and herbs and place in a warm bowl.
2. Meanwhile, cook the pasta as per the instructions and rinse and drain thoroughly.
3. Fold the ricotta into the pasta, then fold in the mackerel. Serve immediately.

DAY 3

LUNCH

Baked Potato

Select a filling from page 121.

DINNER

Lasagna • SERVES 4

4 oz fresh or boxed lasagna, cooked
1 lb lean ground beef or turkey

Red Sauce
1 large onion, finely chopped
1 oz mushrooms, finely chopped
1 red pepper, finely chopped
2 carrots, finely chopped
2 celery sticks, finely chopped
14 oz canned chopped tomatoes
1 tsp chopped fresh, or $1/2$ tsp dried, marjoram
1 tsp chopped fresh, or $1/2$ tsp dried, basil
1 clove garlic, crushed
1 tsp tomato puree

salt and pepper
1 cup meat or vegetable stock

White Sauce
1 cup skim milk
2 oz cornstarch
salt and pepper
$^1/_2$ oz butter
2 oz low-fat cheese, grated

Topping
4 oz cottage cheese

1. Preheat the oven to 325°F.
2. Sauté the vegetables in a heavy-based pan in 1 tbsp of water. Add the canned tomatoes, herbs, garlic, tomato puree, salt and pepper.
3. Add the meat and stock and stir well. Pour the sauce into an ovenproof dish and place in the oven for 1 hour or until the sauce has thickened. Or cook the sauce in a saucepan on top of the stove over low to moderate heat for 20 minutes, stirring regularly.
4. When this is nearly ready, prepare the white sauce. Place 4 tbsp of the milk into a bowl and add the cornstarch, salt and pepper to make a smooth paste. Put the remaining milk and the butter into a pan and heat gently before adding the cheese—do not allow to boil. Pour the warm milk and butter into the cornstarch mixture, mix well and return to the pan. Stir until smooth and thick.
5. Place a layer of the red sauce containing the meat into the bottom of an ovenproof dish, cover with lasagna, then red sauce again. Follow this with a layer of white sauce, another layer of lasagna, then cover completely with the cottage cheese. Place in the oven and bake for approximately 30 minutes at 300°F.

135

Vegetarian Option

Vegetarian Lasagna

Replace the meat with 1 lb mixed vegetables of your choice, such as mushrooms, onions, carrots, peppers (green or red) and zucchini. Prepare as on previous page.

DAY 4

LUNCH

Sandwich

Select a filling from page 121.

DINNER

Chicken Curry • SERVES 4

1 tsp sunflower oil
3 skinless chicken breasts, cubed
1 large onion, chopped
1 clove garlic, crushed
1 large potato, parboiled in the skin and chopped
14 oz canned chopped tomatoes
2 tbsp mango chutney
salt and pepper
1 tsp curry paste (optional)

2 tbsp mild curry powder
1/2 cup chicken stock
3 lemon slices

1. Preheat the oven to 325 °F.
2. Heat the oil gently in a pan, add the meat and brown on both sides. Remove from the pan.
3. Add the onion, garlic and potato to the pan and sauté gently for 2 to 3 minutes, stirring continually. Mix in the tomatoes and chutney and continue to stir. Add salt and pepper to taste.
4. In a separate bowl, mix the curry paste and powder with the chicken stock. Pour over the vegetable mixture in the pan.
5. Replace the chicken, add the lemon slices, cover and place in the oven for 30 to 40 minutes.

Vegetarian Option

Vegetable Curry

Replace the chicken with approximately 10 oz of root vegetables, such as carrots, rutabaga and parsnips, and the chicken stock with vegetable stock. Prepare as above.

DAY 5

LUNCH

Pasta Salad • SERVES 1

1 to 2 oz durum-wheat pasta
1 tbsp fat-free salad dressing
1 apple, chopped
1 small beet, chopped
1 celery stick, chopped
1/2 tsp chopped fresh mint or chives

1. Cook the pasta as per the instructions and drain.
2. Add the dressing to the pasta and stir well.
3. Add the chopped apple, beet and celery and garnish with the mint or chives.

DINNER

Cider Fish Bake • SERVES 4

8 oz leeks, chopped into large chunks
2 carrots, chopped into large chunks
1 clove garlic, crushed
1/2 cup fish or vegetable stock
1 tbsp cornstarch
1/2 cup dry cider
1 lb whiting or monkfish
1 oz low-fat cheese, grated
4 oz fresh bread crumbs
1 tsp sesame seeds
salt and pepper

1. Preheat the oven to 400°F.

2. Place the leeks and carrots in a heavy-based pan and add the garlic. Add 4 tbsp of the stock, cover and cook for 10 minutes or until leeks are soft.
3. Add the remaining stock. Blend the cornstarch with the cider and 2 tbsp of hot vegetable stock taken from the pan. Pour the cider mixture onto the vegetables and bring to a boil gently.
4. Cube the fish and place in an ovenproof dish. Cover with the vegetable mixture.
5. Mix the remaining ingredients together, adding salt and pepper to taste, and sprinkle over the top. Bake for 25 to 30 minutes or until golden brown.

DAY 6

LUNCH

Stuffed Tomato • SERVES 1

2 oz button mushrooms, chopped
1 oz bread crumbs
zest of 1/2 lemon
1 tbsp lemon juice
salt and black pepper
1 tbsp ricotta cheese or cottage cheese
1 large beefsteak tomato

1. Preheat the oven to 275°F.
2. Sauté the mushrooms and add to the bread crumbs.
3. Add the zest and juice of the lemon. Season well with plenty of black pepper and salt to taste and mix everything together with the ricotta or cottage cheese.
4. Scoop out most of the tomato flesh, replace with the filling and bake for 20 minutes.

DINNER

Spaghetti Bolognese • SERVES 4

15 oz spaghetti or fettuccine
1 lb lean ground beef or turkey

Red Sauce
1 large onion, finely chopped
1 oz mushrooms, finely chopped
1 red pepper, finely chopped
2 carrots, finely chopped
2 celery sticks, finely chopped
14 oz canned chopped tomatoes
1/2 tsp marjoram
1 tsp chopped fresh, or 1/2 tsp dried, basil
1 clove garlic, crushed
1 tsp tomato puree
salt and pepper
1 cup meat or vegetable stock

1. Prepare the red sauce as described on pages 134–135.
2. Cook the pasta and rinse and drain it well.
3. Place the pasta in a bowl and top with the red sauce. Serve immediately.

DAY 7

LUNCH

Waldorf Salad • SERVES 1

1 medium red apple, cored and diced
1 tbsp lemon juice, fresh or bottled
2 oz celery, diced
2 tbsp low-fat yogurt or fat-free ricotta cheese
crisp lettuce leaves
4 walnut halves, crushed

1. Toss the diced apple in lemon juice to prevent discoloration. Drain well, then mix with the celery.
2. Add the yogurt or ricotta and toss through the salad, ensuring that all the ingredients are coated with the mixture.
3. Arrange salad on a bed of crisp lettuce leaves and sprinkle with walnuts just before serving.

DINNER

Italian Chicken Casserole • SERVES 4

2 tsp extra-virgin olive oil
4 chicken portions
1 clove garlic, crushed
1 medium onion, chopped
4 oz mushrooms, sliced

14 oz canned chopped tomatoes
1/2 small green pepper, sliced
1/2 red pepper, chopped
1 tbsp chopped fresh parsley, plus a little extra for garnish
1/2 tsp dried thyme
3 tbsp red wine
salt and pepper

1. Preheat the oven to 350°F.
2. Heat the oil gently in a large frying pan, then brown the chicken pieces. Transfer them to an ovenproof casserole dish.
3. Add the garlic, onion and mushrooms to the juices in the pan and sauté gently until tender. Add all the remaining ingredients and bring to a boil, stirring continually.
4. Pour the sauce over the chicken, cover and bake in the oven for 60 minutes. Garnish with the extra chopped parsley.

Vegetarian Option

Vegetable Casserole

Replace the chicken with 6 to 8 oz of vegetables such as eggplants and zucchini and add 14 oz canned, drained borlotti beans. Prepare as above.

DAY 8

LUNCH

Mini Pizza With Mushrooms and Peppers • SERVES 1

6-inch premade pizza crust
4 button mushrooms, chopped
1/2 pepper, chopped
1/2 to 1 level tbsp low-fat cheese, grated

1. Cover the pizza crust with the toppings.
2. Bake according to the instructions on the pizza label.

DINNER

Spicy Fish Dish • SERVES 4

1 tsp olive oil
1 small onion, finely chopped
2 cloves garlic, crushed
1 tbsp fresh gingerroot, finely chopped
4 green cardamom pods
1 tsp ground turmeric
1 tsp ground cumin
2 tbsp ground coriander
1/2 cup plain yogurt
salt and pepper
4 whiting fillets, skinned

1. Preheat the oven to 350°F.
2. Place the oil in a heavy-based pan and add the onion, garlic

and ginger. Cook gently for 2 to 3 minutes, stirring continuously.

3. Remove the pan from the heat. Place the cardamom pods in the mixture. Add the turmeric, cumin and coriander and cook for 2 to 3 minutes, stirring well.
4. Allow the mixture to cool, then stir in the yogurt and seasoning.
5. Place the fish fillets into a large, shallow, ovenproof dish and spread the spicy mixture evenly over each fillet. Cover and bake for 10 minutes.

DAY 9

LUNCH

Baked Potato

Select a filling from page 121.

DINNER

Chicken and Pineapple • SERVES 4

2 tsp olive oil
4 skinless chicken breasts
1 onion, chopped
1 tsp chopped fresh, or $1/2$ tsp dried, thyme
1 large clove garlic, crushed
$1/2$ tsp ground ginger
$1/4$ tsp ground cinnamon
pinch of ground cloves

144

14 oz canned pineapple slices in natural juice, drained
7 oz canned tomatoes
1/3 to 1/2 cup red wine
salt and pepper

1. Preheat the oven to 325°F.
2. Heat the oil and fry the chicken gently on both sides for 3 minutes, stirring to avoid sticking. Transfer to another dish.
3. Add the onion and thyme to the pan and sauté gently until soft. Add the garlic, ginger, cinnamon and cloves and cook for 2 to 3 minutes.
4. Chop the pineapple and mix with the canned tomatoes, wine and seasoning. Add this to the mixture in the pan and cook gently for 2 to 3 minutes.
5. Place some of the mixture in an ovenproof dish, slice the chicken and place on top, followed by the remaining mixture. Cover and bake for approximately 40 minutes.

Vegetarian Option

Chickpea and Mushroom Curry • SERVES 4

2 tsp olive oil
8 oz button mushrooms, quartered
1 small onion, chopped
2 cloves garlic, chopped
1 small piece fresh gingerroot, peeled and chopped
14 oz canned chickpeas, drained
13 oz canned tomatoes
1 tsp ground coriander
1 1/2 oz cashew nuts
1/2 cup vegetable stock
1 tsp mild curry paste

2 tsp hot or medium curry powder

4 tbsp yogurt

2 tbsp chopped fresh coriander (optional)

1. Heat the oil gently in a pan and sauté the mushrooms, onion, garlic and ginger for 2 to 3 minutes.
2. Add the chickpeas, tomatoes, ground coriander and cashew nuts to the mixture.
3. Put the stock, curry paste and curry powder into a bowl. Mix well and pour over the chickpea mixture. Cook gently for 6 to 8 minutes or until the mixture has thickened.
4. Remove from the heat and stir in the yogurt and fresh coriander. Return to a gentle heat for 2 to 3 minutes (do not allow to boil) and serve.

DAY 10

LUNCH

Stir-Fried Vegetables in Pita Bread • SERVES 1

1/2 carrot, chopped

1/3 cucumber, sliced lengthwise

1 oz spring onions, chopped

4 whole baby sweet corn

1/2 oz bean sprouts

generous dash of soy sauce

1 pita bread

1. Cook the vegetables gently in 1 tbsp of water and soy sauce for 3 to 4 minutes.
2. Place the mixture in the pita bread and serve.

DINNER

Piquant Pork • SERVES 4

1 tsp olive oil
4 tender pork cutlets (all fat removed)
1 large onion, chopped
1 clove garlic, crushed
1 tbsp plain or self-rising flour
1 tsp hot paprika
14 oz canned chopped tomatoes
1 tbsp tomato puree
1/2 tbsp brown sugar
2 tbsp wine vinegar
salt and pepper

1. Preheat the oven to 350 °F.
2. Heat the oil gently in a large pan and brown the pork on both sides. Transfer to a large, ovenproof casserole dish.
3. Add the onion and garlic to the pan and sauté for 3 minutes.
4. Remove the pan from the heat, add the flour and paprika and mix well. Return to the heat and continue to stir for 1 minute.
5. Add the tomatoes, puree, sugar, wine vinegar, and salt and pepper to taste. Stir well as you bring to a boil. Pour over the pork, cover and bake for 1 hour.

Vegetarian Option

Vegetables in Piquant Sauce • SERVES 4

Replace the pork with 5 oz cauliflower florets and 5 oz broccoli florets. Prepare the sauce as above and place the cauliflower and broccoli in an ovenproof dish. Stir 1 oz whole almonds into the sauce and pour it over the broccoli and cauliflower. Cover and cook for 30 minutes.

DAY 11

LUNCH

Sandwich

Select a filling from page 121.

DINNER

Stir-Fried Beef, Chicken or Turkey in Black Bean Sauce

1 tsp sesame oil
12 oz beef, chicken or turkey, very thinly sliced
3 spring onions, chopped
1/2 red pepper, sliced
1 carrot, thinly sliced
1/2 celery stick, thinly sliced
2 oz mushrooms, thinly sliced
1 small onion, sliced
1 clove garlic
1 tsp ground ginger
2 tbsp soy sauce
1 tsp cornstarch
1 tbsp sherry
1 to 2 tbsp black bean sauce
1 cup meat or vegetable stock

1. Heat the oil gently and stir-fry the meat for 2 to 3 minutes,
   stirring continuously. Remove from the pan.

2. Sauté all the vegetables gently for 2 to 3 minutes, remove and place with the meat.
3. Add the garlic, ginger and soy sauce to the pan and cook for 1 to 2 minutes, stirring constantly.
4. In a separate bowl, mix the cornstarch and sherry to a smooth paste. Stir in the black bean sauce.
5. Add the stock to the ginger and garlic in the pan and bring to a boil. Take 2 tbsp of this hot liquid and add to the cornstarch mixture. Pour this cornstarch mixture into the pan and stir until thickened. Return the meat and vegetables to the pan and heat thoroughly.

Vegetarian Option

Stir-Fried Vegetables in Black Bean Sauce

Replace the meat with 1 lb of vegetables, such as bean sprouts, snow peas, carrots, cucumber, spring onions, celery, baby sweet corn and red pepper. Prepare as above, but when stir-frying your chosen vegetables, add 4 oz chickpeas to the mixture.

DAY 12

LUNCH

Beans on Toast • SERVES 1

2 thick slices of toast (without butter) with a small can of baked beans.

DINNER

Fish Plaki • SERVES 4

1 1/2 lb fresh or frozen trout, cod or haddock, skinned
1 tbsp olive oil
1 large onion, thinly sliced
1 clove garlic, crushed
4 tbsp chopped fresh parsley
14 oz canned chopped tomatoes
1 tbsp lemon juice
salt and pepper
4 lemon slices

1. Preheat the oven to 350°F.
2. Cut the fish into 4 portions and place in a large, shallow, ovenproof dish.
3. Heat the oil gently before adding the onion, garlic and parsley. Sauté for 2 to 3 minutes. Add the tomatoes, lemon juice and seasoning and bring to a boil.
4. Pour over the fish and place the lemon slices on top. Cover and cook in the oven for 25 minutes. Remove the cover and bake for another 10 to 15 minutes.

DAY 13

LUNCH

Sandwich

Select a filling from page 121.

DINNER

Chili con Carne • SERVES 4

1 tbsp olive oil
1 clove garlic, crushed
1 medium onion, chopped
4 oz mushrooms, chopped
1 red pepper, sliced
14 oz canned chopped tomatoes
1 lb lean ground beef
1 to 2 tbsp tomato puree
15 oz canned red kidney beans
1 tbsp chili powder
1 tsp chili sauce
salt and pepper

1. Heat the oil gently in a pan and add the garlic. Sauté the onion, mushrooms and pepper for 2 to 3 minutes, stirring continuously. Add the canned tomatoes and cook for another minute. Remove and place in a bowl.
2. Fry the meat gently in the vegetable juices for 3 to 4 minutes, stirring continually. Replace the vegetables and mix in with the meat before adding the puree and the kidney beans.

3. Mix the chili powder and chili sauce together in a separate cup, then stir into the mixture, adding salt and pepper to taste. Cover and cook for 30 minutes on a very low heat.

Vegetarian Option

Vegetarian Chili

Replace the ground beef with 1 lb of vegetables, such as mashed rutabaga, grated carrot and eggplant. Prepare as above.

DAY 14

LUNCH

Curried Parsnip Soup • SERVES 4 • CAN BE FROZEN

3 parsnips, chopped
1 large onion, chopped
1 tbsp curry powder or sauce
1/2 cup milk
1/2 cup water
chopped fresh coriander (optional), to taste

1. Place the parsnips and onion in a heavy-based pan with the curry powder or sauce, stir well and cook for 2 to 3 minutes in 1 tbsp of water.
2. Add the milk and water and cook on a low heat for another 45 minutes. Puree and serve. The coriander can be added for extra flavor.

DINNER

Autumn Pie • SERVES 4

1 tsp olive oil
1 large onion, chopped
2 large carrots, cut into thick sticks
4 oz zucchini, cut into thick sticks
13 oz canned chopped tomatoes
10 oz lean ground beef, fried in a nonstick pan and drained of fat
salt and pepper
3 tbsp frozen peas
12 oz potatoes, peeled
3 tbsp fresh bread crumbs

1. Preheat the oven to 325°F.
2. Heat the oil gently and sauté the onion for 2 to 3 minutes. Add the carrots, zucchini and tomatoes and cook for an additional 2 to 3 minutes. Remove from the pan and place in a bowl.
3. Sauté the ground beef gently until browned, stirring constantly. Replace the vegetables and continue to cook. Season to taste, add the peas and leave on a low heat for 10 minutes.
4. Meanwhile, boil and mash the potatoes. Place the meat in an ovenproof dish, spread the potato on top and sprinkle with the bread crumbs. Bake in the oven for 50 to 60 minutes.

Vegetarian Option

Leek and Bean Macaroni • SERVES 4

12 oz whole-wheat macaroni
1 tsp olive oil
12 oz leeks, thinly sliced
14 oz canned mixed beans
1 tsp coarse-grain mustard
4 oz cottage cheese

White Sauce
1 cup skim milk
2 oz cornstarch
salt and pepper
$1/2$ oz butter
2 oz low-fat cheese, grated

1. Preheat the oven to 425°F.
2. Cook the macaroni as per the instructions on the package, rinse and drain.
3. Heat the oil in a heavy-based pan and sauté the leeks for 3 to 4 minutes.
4. Remove the pan from the heat and add the beans, leaving 1 tbsp of the bean water to mix together with the mustard. Add this to the leek-and-bean mixture.
5. Prepare the white sauce as on page 135. Mix the macaroni in with the white sauce and add this to the bean mixture. Stir well and remove from the pan and place in a large oven-proof dish. Top with the cottage cheese and bake for 20 minutes.

DAY 15

LUNCH

Sandwich

Select a filling from page 121.

DINNER

Chili Chicken With Orange • SERVES 4

2 onions, sliced
1 red pepper, sliced
4 oz mushrooms, sliced
14 oz canned chili beans
13 oz canned tomatoes
salt and pepper
2 tsp tomato puree
1 sprig of parsley, chopped
$1/2$ tsp chili powder
4 chicken breasts
2 oranges

1. Place the onions, pepper and mushrooms in a casserole pan with a thick bottom. Sweat the vegetables for 5 minutes, stirring constantly.
2. Add the chili beans, tomatoes, salt, pepper, tomato puree, parsley and chili powder.
3. Grill the chicken pieces for about 2 minutes, to seal just the outside.

4. Squeeze the juice from an orange into the vegetable mixture, then add the chicken pieces. Top with a layer of sliced orange from the remaining orange. Cover the casserole and cook for 1¹/₂ to 2 hours over a low heat or until the sauce is thick. Serve with rice.

Vegetarian Option

Vegetables in Chili and Orange Sauce

Replace the chicken with 1 lb of root vegetables such as rutabaga and carrots. Prepare as above, but add 4 oz of cooked lentils 10 minutes before serving.

DAY 16

LUNCH

Vegetable and Bean Soup • SERVES 4

1 tbsp olive oil
1 large onion, roughly chopped
1 large parsnip, peeled and roughly chopped
1 large carrot, peeled and roughly chopped
1 large potato, peeled and roughly chopped
2 zucchini, thinly sliced
1 to 2 cups vegetable stock
1 to 2 tsp mild curry paste
1 clove garlic, crushed

15 oz canned red kidney beans, drained and rinsed
15 oz canned black-eyed peas, drained and rinsed
salt and pepper
3 tbsp chopped fresh coriander

1. Heat the oil gently and sauté the vegetables for 3 to 4 minutes.
2. In a separate bowl, mix together the stock, curry paste and garlic and pour this onto the vegetables. Stir and simmer for 25 to 30 minutes or until the vegetables are tender. (You can puree the mixture at this stage if a smoother texture is preferred.)
3. Mix in the beans and season to taste, before adding the coriander. Simmer for 10 minutes and serve.

DINNER

Tuna Salad • SERVES 4

12 oz spinach pasta
1 oz pine nuts or almonds
1/2 lb tomatoes, chopped into wedges
14 oz canned tuna fish in spring water
4 tbsp chopped fresh basil
Italian garlic dressing (fat-free)

1. Cook the pasta as per the instructions, rinse and drain.
2. Brown the nuts on a baking tray in the oven.
3. Drain the tuna fish and mix everything together with the dressing. Serve immediately.

DAY 17

LUNCH

Tasty Tomatoes on Toast • SERVES 1

1 slice thickly cut bread
7 oz canned tomatoes
pinch of fresh basil
1 oz low-fat cottage cheese

1. Brown the bread on one side and mix the tomatoes and basil together before spreading on the other side.
2. Place the cottage cheese on top of the tomatoes and broil for 2 to 3 minutes.

DINNER

Shepherd's Pie • SERVES 4

12 oz to 1 lb lean ground beef
1 1/2 lb potatoes

Red Sauce
1 large onion, finely chopped
1 oz mushrooms, finely chopped
1 red pepper, finely chopped
2 carrots, finely chopped
2 celery sticks, finely chopped
14 oz canned chopped tomatoes
1/2 tsp marjoram
1 tsp chopped fresh, or 1/2 tsp dried, basil

1 clove garlic, crushed
1 tsp tomato puree
salt and pepper
1 cup meat or vegetable stock

1. Preheat the oven to 425°F.
2. Prepare the red sauce as on pages 134–135 and pour the cooked red sauce containing the meat into a deep ovenproof dish.
3. Cook and mash the potatoes and cover the red sauce with them. Place in the oven for 30 minutes or until the potato browns.

Vegetarian Option

Vegetarian Shepherd's Pie • SERVES 4

Replace the meat with approximately 1 1/2 lb canned mixed, cannellini or kidney beans. Prepare as above.

DAY 18

LUNCH

Mini Pizza With Sweet Corn and Green Beans • SERVES 1

6-inch premade pizza crust
1 to 2 tbsp sweet corn
1 to 2 tbsp canned green beans

Prepare as on page 143. If you wish, top with 1/2 to 1 level tbsp of low-fat cottage cheese.

DINNER

Beef Stew With Cider • SERVES 4

1 lb rump steak, cut into cubes
1 large onion, roughly chopped
2 carrots, roughly chopped
2 turnips, roughly chopped
2 celery sticks, roughly chopped
2 cups meat or vegetable stock
1 tbsp flour, seasoned with salt and pepper
1/2 cup cider

1. Preheat the oven to 300°F.
2. Place the meat and vegetables in a pan and add 4 tbsp of the stock. Cook for 5 to 6 minutes and remove from the heat.
3. In a separate bowl, mix the flour and 2 tbsp of stock into a paste. Pour the remaining stock over the meat and vegetables, stirring well.
4. Pour the flour mixture back into the pan with the meat and vegetables. Stir well and cook until the sauce thickens. Add the cider and put the mixture into an ovenproof dish, cover and bake for 1 to 1 1/2 hours.

Vegetarian Option

Vegetable and Nut Stir-Fry • SERVES 4

1 tsp sesame oil
4 oz baby sweet corn
1 large red pepper, cut into strips
5 oz snow peas
1 bunch spring onions, shredded
10 oz button mushrooms, sliced
1 oz fresh gingerroot, grated
4 tbsp soy sauce
$1/2$ tbsp honey
1 tbsp cornstarch
1 tbsp tomato puree
1 cup vegetable stock
8 oz bean sprouts
2 oz split cashew nuts

1. Heat the oil in a wok or large frying pan. Add the corn, pepper and snow peas. Then add the onions, mushrooms and ginger and stir-fry for 2 to 3 minutes. Remove the vegetables from the pan and place in a bowl.
2. Put the soy sauce and honey into the pan.
3. In a separate bowl, combine the cornstarch, tomato puree and 1 tbsp of the vegetable stock. Mix these to a smooth paste.
4. Heat the soy sauce and the honey and pour onto the cornstarch mixture, then pour this mixture back into the pan and cook to a smooth paste.
5. Stir in the bean sprouts and cook for 2 minutes. Add the vegetables and nuts and cook for another 5 minutes. Serve immediately.

DAY 19

LUNCH

Baked Potato

Select a filling from page 121.

DINNER

Crunchy Fish Dish • SERVES 4

2 oz fresh bread crumbs
1 tsp mustard powder
4 tbsp bran flakes or cornflakes, crushed
1 tbsp low-fat cheese, grated
1 tbsp chopped fresh parsley
1 tsp dried thyme
zest of 1 lemon
1 tsp olive oil and a little lemon juice, mixed together
1 1/2 lb cod fillet, skinned and cut into 4 pieces
salt and pepper

1. Preheat the oven to 350°F.
2. Mix together the bread crumbs, mustard, bran flakes or cornflakes, low-fat cheese, parsley, thyme and lemon zest.
3. Brush an ovenproof dish with the olive oil and lemon juice and lay the pieces of fish in it. Brush the fish with the same mixture.
4. Coat each piece of fish with the bread crumb mixture, cover and bake for 30 minutes or until the topping is brown and the fish cooked. Salt and pepper to taste.

DAY 20

LUNCH

Tomato and Rice Soup • SERVES 4 • CAN BE FROZEN

1 large onion, finely chopped
1 large carrot, finely chopped
14 oz canned chopped tomatoes
1 tsp olive oil
3 cups chicken or vegetable stock
$1/4$ tsp dried marjoram
salt and pepper
2 tbsp uncooked brown rice
1 tbsp fresh parsley, chopped

1. Place the onion, carrot and tomatoes in a pan with the olive oil and sauté for 5 minutes.
2. Add all the remaining ingredients, except the rice and parsley, and bring to a boil. Cover and simmer for 30 minutes.
3. Add the rice and simmer for an additional 12 minutes. Stir in the parsley just before serving.

DINNER

Chicken in Barbecue Sauce • SERVES 4

1 tsp olive oil
1 large onion, chopped
4 skinless chicken breasts
14 oz canned chopped tomatoes
1 tsp English mustard
1 tbsp brown sugar
2 tbsp wine vinegar
2 tbsp Worcestershire sauce
1/4 tsp garlic powder
1/4 tsp salt
1 tsp chili powder
2 tsp tomato puree

1. Heat the oil and sauté the onion until golden brown. Add the chicken breasts and fry gently for approximately 5 minutes or until browned.
2. Add all the remaining ingredients and bring to a boil, stirring continuously. Cover and simmer for 25 minutes.
3. Either serve as is or remove the chicken and puree the sauce to serve with the chicken. (This barbecue sauce can also be used as a topping for baked potatoes.)

Vegetarian Option

Zucchini and Carrot Loaf • SERVES 4

1 small onion
1 oz nuts (almonds or other)
4 oz zucchini, grated
4 oz carrots, grated
1 oz oats (not instant)
1 tbsp tomato puree
1/4 tsp dried mixed herbs
salt and pepper

1. Preheat the oven to 350 °F.
2. Sauté the onion gently for 5 minutes. Add the nuts, zucchini and carrots and cook for another 5 minutes.
3. Stir in the remaining ingredients and spoon the mixture into a 2-lb nonstick loaf pan, pressing down well.
4. Bake near the top of the oven for approximately 25 minutes or until brown. Allow to cool for 3 to 5 minutes before turning out onto a plate and serving.

DAY 21

LUNCH

Sandwich

Select a filling from page 121.

DINNER

Sweet Pork or Chicken Pot • SERVES 4

1 tsp olive oil
1 lb lean, boneless pork or chicken, cubed
1 red pepper, sliced
1 green pepper, sliced
1 onion, chopped
1 oz potatoes, sliced
1 tbsp tomato puree
$1/2$ cup white wine
3 tbsp pineapple juice
1 sprig of fresh thyme
salt and pepper
1 cup chicken stock
2 tbsp cornstarch
4 oz sweet corn
4 oz pineapple, diced
1 tbsp chopped fresh parsley

1. Heat the oil gently and sauté the meat, peppers, onion and potatoes. Stir continually and cook for 5 to 6 minutes.
2. Add the tomato puree, white wine, pineapple juice, thyme, salt and pepper and bring to a boil.
3. Use 4 tbsp of the stock with the cornstarch to make a smooth paste and add the remaining stock to the vegetables and meat.

166

4. Heat the meat and vegetable mixture gently for 20 minutes. Stir in the cornstarch mixture and simmer for 3 minutes or until the sauce has thickened.
5. Add the sweet corn, pineapple and parsley. Stir and simmer for 3 minutes.

Vegetarian Option

Spicy Peas and Potatoes • SERVES 4

1 tsp olive oil
2 large onions, chopped
1 clove garlic, crushed
6 green cardamom pods
2 tbsp cumin seeds
1 oz fresh gingerroot, peeled and chopped
1 green chili, seeded and chopped
1 bay leaf
2 lb potatoes, cubed
1 tsp turmeric
salt and pepper
$1/2$ cup vegetable stock
12 oz frozen peas
$1/2$ cup plain yogurt
2 oz chopped nuts (preferably almonds)

1. Heat the oil gently in a saucepan. Add the onions, garlic, cardamom pods, cumin, ginger, chili and bay leaf to the pan and sauté for 10 minutes, stirring continuously.
2. Add the potatoes, turmeric and seasoning and pour in the stock. Cover and simmer for 15 minutes.
3. Stir in the peas and simmer for another 10 to 15 minutes or until the potatoes are soft.
4. Add the yogurt while still heating gently (do not boil). Sprinkle with the chopped nuts just before serving.

DAY 22

LUNCH

Tomato Soup • SERVES 4 TO 6 • CAN BE FROZEN

1 tsp olive oil
1 medium onion, chopped
1 medium carrot, chopped
1 celery stick, chopped
14 oz canned chopped tomatoes
3 cups chicken or vegetable stock
1 medium potato, chopped
2 tsp tomato puree
pinch of salt and pepper
$1/2$ cup skim milk

1. Heat the oil gently in a large pan, add the onion, carrot and celery and sauté for 10 minutes.
2. Add the tomatoes, stock, potato, puree and seasoning. Cover and simmer for 45 minutes.
3. Puree the mixture, stir in the milk and reheat to serve.

DINNER

Moussaka • SERVES 4

2 medium eggplants, sliced
salt
2 medium onions, sliced
1 lb ground beef
13 oz canned tomatoes

1 tbsp chopped parsley
pinch of nutmeg
1 clove garlic
pepper
2 tbsp tomato puree
1 cup plain low-fat yogurt
1 tbsp cottage cheese

1. Sprinkle the eggplant with salt and leave for 30 minutes. Preheat the oven to 300 °F.
2. Dry sauté the slices of eggplant for 5 minutes and then remove from the heat.
3. Sauté the onions and beef and add the tomatoes, parsley, nutmeg, garlic, salt, pepper and tomato puree. Simmer for 30 minutes.
4. Place alternate layers of eggplant and meat sauce in an oven-proof dish until the top layer is eggplant.
5. Mix the yogurt and cottage cheese together and pour over the eggplant. Bake for 20 minutes and broil just before serving to brown. Serve with whole-wheat bread and salad.

Vegetarian Option

Vegetarian Moussaka

Prepare as above, but replace the beef with 1 lb root vegetables, cooked and mashed.

DAY 23

LUNCH

Baked Potato

Select a filling from page 121.

DINNER

Smoked Haddock Loaf • SERVES 4

1¹/₂ lb smoked haddock or cod
¹/₂ cup milk
salt and pepper
2 eggs
1 sprig of parsley, chopped

White Sauce
1 oz cornstarch
1 oz butter
2 oz low-fat Cheddar cheese, grated

1. Preheat the oven to 300°F.
2. Place the fish in a dish with the milk, add salt and pepper to taste and bake for approximately 20 minutes until flaking. Separate the eggs and add the flaked fish to the egg yolks.
3. Prepare the white sauce as described on page 135, but use the milk from the cooked fish. Add the cheese, parsley and the fish mixture.
4. Whisk the egg whites until very stiff and fold into the fish mixture. Place in a 2-lb loaf pan lined with foil (or use a mold) and bake for 30 minutes.
5. Turn out onto a plate and slice.

170

DAY 24

LUNCH

Vegetable Rice • SERVES 1

8 oz frozen rice with peas and mushrooms
Carrots, sliced, as desired
Sweet corn, as desired

1. Sauté everything gently with water (not oil as directed on some rice labels) until soft.
2. Serve immediately.

DINNER

Steamed Ginger Chicken • SERVES 4

4 skinless chicken breasts
4 tbsp sherry
3 tbsp soy sauce
8 spring onions, cut into small slices
2 oz fresh gingerroot, peeled and chopped

1. Place the chicken in an ovenproof dish.
2. Mix the sherry and soy sauce together and add the onions and ginger.
3. Spoon the mixture over the chicken, cover and marinate for several hours (or overnight) in the refrigerator.
4. Turn the chicken breasts over and cover the dish with foil. Bake at 300 °F for 45 minutes or until the chicken is tender.

Vegetarian Option

Stuffed Mushrooms • SERVES 4

1 tsp olive oil
1 clove garlic, crushed
1 small onion, very finely chopped
3 oz fresh bread crumbs
2 pineapple rings, chopped
8 oz cottage cheese
salt and pepper
grated nutmeg
8 large, flat mushrooms, stalks removed

1. Preheat the oven to 400°F.
2. Heat the oil gently in a pan and add the garlic and onion. Stir-fry until the onion is soft, then add the bread crumbs.
3. Stir in the pineapple and cottage cheese and add salt, pepper and nutmeg to taste.
4. Place the mushrooms in an ovenproof dish and fill each one with the stuffing. Bake for 20 to 25 minutes.

DAY 25

LUNCH

Pizza Bread and Tuna Fish • SERVES 1

Prepare as on page 143, but add 1 oz of tuna fish.

DINNER

Fruity Chicken Biryani • SERVES 4

1 tsp olive oil
1 oz onion, finely chopped
1 clove garlic, crushed
1 red pepper, chopped
3/4 to 1 cup chicken stock
1/2 tsp turmeric
1 tbsp curry paste
10 oz skinless, boneless chicken, cubed
2 oz apricots
1 oz raisins
3 oz long-grain rice
2 tsp low-sugar apricot jam
pinch of salt and pepper
1 tbsp flaked almonds
6 tbsp plain low-fat yogurt
2 tbsp cucumber, finely chopped

1. Heat the oil gently and add the onion, garlic and red pepper and cook for 2 to 3 minutes.
2. Mix the chicken stock, turmeric and curry paste in a separate bowl. Pour over the onion mixture.
3. Add the chicken, simmer for 8 to 10 minutes, then add the apricots, raisins, rice, and jam. Salt and pepper to taste. Bring to a boil, stir and cover. Simmer and cook for 20 minutes or until the rice and chicken are tender.
4. Transfer to a serving dish and top with the flaked almonds. Mix the yogurt and cucumber together to add on the side.

Vegetarian Option

Vegetable Biryani

Replace the chicken with 1 lb fruity root vegetables, such as parsnips, rutabaga, squash and pumpkin, and replace the chicken stock with vegetable stock. Prepare as above.

DAY 26

LUNCH

Sandwich

Select a filling from page 121.

DINNER

Kedgeree • SERVES 4

8 oz long-grain brown rice
1 egg
10 oz smoked haddock
1 tbsp fresh parsley, chopped
juice of 1/2 lemon
salt and pepper
1/2 oz butter or 2 oz ricotta cheese

1. Cook the rice as usual, drain and rinse.
2. Hard-boil the egg, chop it into pieces and add, along with the haddock, parsley and lemon, to the rice.
3. When ready to serve, add the butter or ricotta cheese. Reheat in the microwave or oven and stir well. Salt and pepper to taste

DAY 27

LUNCH

Baked Potato

Select a filling from page 121.

DINNER

Lemon Chicken • SERVES 4

4 skinless chicken breasts, cut into strips
1 tsp sesame oil
$1/2$ tsp garlic, finely chopped
1 tsp fresh gingerroot
1 red pepper, sliced
2 oz mushrooms, sliced
5 spring onions, chopped
1 dried red chili or $1/4$ tsp chili powder
1 tsp cornstarch, blended with 1 tsp water
2 tsp dry sherry or rice wine
2 tsp reduced-sodium soy sauce
1 to 2 tbsp fresh lemon juice
2 tsp brown sugar
zest of 1 lemon
$1/3$ to $1/2$ cup water or chicken stock

1. Sauté the chicken gently in the sesame oil and garlic for 2 to 3 minutes. Remove from the pan.
2. Add the vegetables, chili and ginger to the pan and sauté for 2 to 3 minutes. Remove from the pan.
3. Put the cornstarch and the sherry or rice wine into a separate bowl and mix to make a paste.
4. Put the soy sauce, lemon juice, sugar and lemon zest in the

pan, simmer for 1 minute, then pour onto the cornstarch mixture. Stir well, then return to the pan to make a thick sauce. Add the chicken stock or water.

5. Return the chicken to the pan and cook for 5 minutes. Add the vegetables and cook for another 5 minutes.

Vegetarian Option

Lentil and Zucchini Bake • SERVES 4

1 tsp olive oil
1 onion, finely chopped
1 clove garlic, crushed
1 bay leaf
2 celery sticks, thinly sliced
2 carrots, diced
8 oz red lentils
2 cups vegetable stock
1 lb zucchini, sliced
salt and pepper
1 oz Cheddar cheese, grated
1 oz fresh bread crumbs
pinch of cayenne pepper

1. Heat the oil gently and add the onion, garlic, bay leaf, celery and carrots. Sauté for 2 to 3 minutes, add the lentils and stock and bring to a boil.
2. Stir, cover and simmer for 20 to 25 minutes or until the lentils are soft.
3. Preheat the oven to 350 °F.
4. Lay half of the zucchini in an ovenproof dish, cover with the lentil mixture, top with the remaining zucchini and sprinkle with seasoning.
5. Mix the cheese, bread crumbs and cayenne pepper together and spread over the zucchini. Bake for 30 to 35 minutes.

DAY 28

LUNCH

Sandwich

Select a filling from page 121.

DINNER

Meat Loaf • SERVES 4

5 slices bread, grated into crumbs
3/4 lb ground beef
2 tsp tomato puree
1 bouillon cube
3 carrots, grated
1 small onion, finely chopped
1/2 red pepper, finely chopped
1 sprig of parsley, chopped
salt and pepper
1 egg

1. Preheat the oven to 350°F and line a 1-lb loaf pan with foil.
2. Put all the ingredients into a bowl and mix.
3. Place the mixture in the loaf pan and bake for 30 minutes.

Vegetarian Option

Vegetable Casserole • SERVES 4 TO 6

2 tsp olive oil
13 oz onions, chopped
2 cloves garlic, crushed
2 green peppers, sliced
13 oz zucchini, chopped
2 medium eggplants, chopped
7 oz mushrooms, sliced
14 oz canned tomatoes
3 oz tomato puree
2 bay leaves
1 tbsp fresh parsley, chopped
1 tsp fresh marjoram, chopped
1 tsp fresh thyme, chopped
salt and pepper
1 cup water or vegetable stock
13 oz potatoes, peeled and thinly sliced

1. Preheat the oven to 350°F.
2. Heat the oil in the pan and add the onions, garlic, peppers, zucchini, eggplant and mushrooms. Sauté gently for 5 minutes.
3. Add the tomatoes, puree, herbs and seasoning. Mix well and pour in the stock.
4. Arrange the potatoes on the top, cover and bake for 1 hour. Remove the lid and bake for another 30 minutes.

AFTER 28 DAYS—WHAT HAPPENS NOW?

As you have read through this book, you have learned a lot about how your body works and what it needs to function properly. You have also learned about what it doesn't need to function—and that some foods can be quite harmful to your body and can make you gain weight.

If you have followed this plan for 28 days, you could simply start again. After all, the recipes are so delicious that you could carry on cooking these meals forever. I hope that you have also learned enough to be able to adapt some of your own favorite recipes that were not included in the book. Remember: A diet isn't something you go on and then come off. If you have made the important decision to watch what you eat, it doesn't stop here. In fact, this is just the beginning.

If you have followed the recipes and done the exercises, then you will be feeling fitter by now, and you will have more energy and feel less lethargic and generally healthier. Perhaps people are starting to comment on how well you look—you will certainly feel much better. All the good work you have been doing over the past month must be carried on until it becomes a way of life—not a hardship, but a way of living life to the fullest. If you look after your body, it adds years to your life and life to your years. Go for it.

Index

181